Cytology

Editor

AMY L. MacNEILL

VETERINARY CLINICS OF NORTH AMERICA: SMALL ANIMAL PRACTICE

www.vetsmall.theclinics.com

January 2017 • Volume 47 • Number 1

ELSEVIER

1600 John F. Kennedy Boulevard ● Suite 1800 ● Philadelphia, Pennsylvania, 19103-2899
http://www.vetsmall.theclinics.com

VETERINARY CLINICS OF NORTH AMERICA: SMALL ANIMAL PRACTICE Volume 47, Number 1
January 2017 ISSN 0195-5616, ISBN-13: 978-0-323-48274-5

Editor: Katie Pfaff
Developmental Editor: Meredith Clinton

Veterinary Clinics of North America: Small Animal Practice (ISSN 0195-5616) is published bimonthly by Elsevier Inc., 360 Park Avenue South, New York, NY 10010-1710. Months of issue are January, March, May, July, September, and November. Business and Editorial Offices: 1600 John F. Kennedy Blvd., Ste. 1800, Philadelphia, PA 19103-2899. Customer Service Office: 3251 Riverport Lane, Maryland Heights, MO 63043. Periodicals postage paid at New York, NY and additional mailing offices. Subscription prices are $319.00 per year (domestic individuals), $598.00 per year (domestic institutions), $100.00 per year (domestic students/residents), $422.00 per year (Canadian individuals), $743.00 per year (Canadian institutions), $469.00 per year (international individuals), $743.00 per year (international institutions), and $220.00 per year (international and Canadian students/residents). To receive student/resident rate, orders must be accompained by name of affiliated institution, date of term, and the *signature* of program/residency coordinator on institution letterhead. Orders will be billed at individual rate until proof of status is received. Foreign air speed delivery is included in all *Clinics* subscription prices. All prices are subject to change without notice. **POSTMASTER:** Send address changes to *Veterinary Clinics of North America: Small Animal Practice*, Elsevier Health Sciences Division, Subscription Customer Service, 3251 Riverport Lane, Maryland Heights, MO 63043. Customer Service (orders, claims, online, change of address): Elsevier Periodicals Customer Service, Elsevier Health Sciences Division Subscription **Customer Service 3251 Riverport Lane Maryland Heights, MO 63043. Tel: 1-800-654-2452 (U.S. and Canada); 314-447-8871 (outside U.S. and Canada). Fax: 314-447-8029. E-mail: journalscustomerservice-usa@elsevier.com (for print support); journalsonlinesupport-usa@elsevier.com (for online support).**

Reprints. For copies of 100 or more of articles in this publication, please contact the Commercial Reprints Department, Elsevier Inc., 360 Park Avenue South, New York, NY 10010-1710. Tel.: 212-633-3874; Fax: 212-633-3820; E-mail: reprints@elsevier.com.

Veterinary Clinics of North America: Small Animal Practice is also published in Japanese by Inter Zoo Publishing Co., Ltd., Aoyama Crystal-Bldg 5F, 3-5-12 Kitaaoyama, Minato-ku, Tokyo 107-0061, Japan.

Veterinary Clinics of North America: Small Animal Practice is covered in *Current Contents/Agriculture, Biology and Environmental Sciences, Science Citation Index, ASCA, MEDLINE/PubMed (Index Medicus), Excerpta Medica,* and *BIOSIS.*

Contributors

EDITOR

AMY L. MacNEILL, DVM, PhD, DACVP
Diplomate, American College of Veterinary Pathologists (Clinical Pathology);
Associate Professor, Clinical Pathology Section; Residency Coordinator, Department of
Microbiology, Immunology, and Pathology, College of Veterinary Medicine and
Biomedical Sciences, Colorado State University, Fort Collins, Colorado

AUTHORS

PAUL R. AVERY, VMD, PhD
Diplomate, American College of Veterinary Pathologists (Clinical Pathology);
Associate Professor, Department of Microbiology, Immunology, and Pathology, College of
Veterinary Medicine and Biomedical Sciences, Colorado State University, Fort Collins,
Colorado

ANNE M. BARGER, DVM, MS
Diplomate, American College of Veterinary Pathologists; Clinical Professor, Pathobiology
Department, University of Illinois, Urbana, Illinois

ANDREA A. BOHN, DVM, PhD
Diplomate, American College of Veterinary Pathologists (Clinical Pathology);
Associate Professor, Department of Microbiology, Immunology, and Pathology, College of
Veterinary Medicine and Biomedical Sciences, Colorado State University, Fort Collins,
Colorado

JOHN W. HARVEY, DVM, PhD
Diplomate, American College of Veterinary Pathology; Professor Emeritus, Department of
Physiological Sciences, College of Veterinary Medicine, University of Florida, Gainesville,
Florida

MARK C. JOHNSON, DVM
Diplomate, American College of Veterinary Pathologists; Clinical Associate Professor,
Department of Veterinary Pathobiology, College of Veterinary Medicine and Biomedical
Sciences, Texas A&M University, College Station, Texas

AMY L. MacNEILL, DVM, PhD
Diplomate, American College of Veterinary Pathologists (Clinical Pathology);
Associate Professor, Clinical Pathology Section; Residency Coordinator, Department of
Microbiology, Immunology, and Pathology, College of Veterinary Medicine and
Biomedical Sciences, Colorado State University, Fort Collins, Colorado

CAITLYN R. MARTINEZ, DVM
Postdoctoral Researcher, Department of Microbiology, Immunology, and Pathology,
College of Veterinary Medicine and Biomedical Sciences, Colorado State University,
Fort Collins, Colorado

A RUSSELL MOORE, DVM, MS
Diplomate, American College of Veterinary Pathologists (Clinical Pathology); Assistant Professor, Department of Microbiology, Immunology, and Pathology, College of Veterinary Medicine and Biomedical Sciences, Colorado State University, Fort Collins, Colorado

ALEXANDRA N. MYERS, DVM
Clinical Pathology Resident, Department of Veterinary Pathobiology, College of Veterinary Medicine and Biomedical Sciences, Texas A&M University, College Station, Texas

CHRISTINE S. OLVER, DVM, PhD
Diplomate, American College of Veterinary Pathologists; Department of Microbiology, Immunology, and Pathology, College of Veterinary Medicine and Biomedical Sciences, Colorado State University, Fort Collins, Colorado

LAUREN B. RADAKOVICH, DVM
Department of Microbiology, Immunology, and Pathology, College of Veterinary Medicine and Biomedical Sciences, Colorado State University, Fort Collins, Colorado

EMILY D. ROUT, DVM
Clinical Pathology Resident, Department of Microbiology, Immunology, and Pathology, College of Veterinary Medicine and Biomedical Sciences, Colorado State University, Fort Collins, Colorado

KELLY S. SANTANGELO, DVM, PhD
Diplomate, American College of Veterinary Pathologists; Assistant Professor, Department of Microbiology, Immunology, and Pathology, College of Veterinary Medicine and Biomedical Sciences, Colorado State University, Fort Collins, Colorado

SARAH B. SHROPSHIRE, DVM
Diplomate, American College of Veterinary Internal Medicine (Small Animal); PhD Candidate, Department of Clinical Sciences, College of Veterinary Medicine and Biomedical Sciences, Colorado State University, Fort Collins, Colorado

NICOLE I. STACY, DVM, Dr med vet
Diplomate, American College of Veterinary Pathology; Clinical Assistant Professor, Department of Large Animal Clinical Sciences, College of Veterinary Medicine, University of Florida, Gainesville, Florida

CRAIG A. THOMPSON, DVM
Diplomate, American College of Veterinary Pathologists (Clinical Pathology); Clinical Assistant Professor, Clinical Pathology; Residency Coordinator, Department of Comparative Pathobiology, College of Veterinary Medicine, Purdue University, West Lafayette, Indiana

LINDA M. VAP, DVM
Diplomate, American College of Veterinary Pathologists (Clinical Pathology); Assistant Professor, Department of Microbiology, Immunology, and Pathology, College of Veterinary Medicine and Biomedical Sciences, Colorado State University, Fort Collins, Colorado

Contents

General principles and techniques for collection, preparation, and staining of cytologic samples in the general practice setting are reviewed. Tips for collection of digital images are also discussed.

Iron, particularly hemosiderin, is a commonly observed pigment in cytology. Many pigments appear green to blue to black, making differentiation of pigment types difficult. While cytologic clues such as erythrophagia can help determine whether pigment is iron, Perl's Prussian Blue stain is used to highlight iron when these clues are not present. Other special stains can identify similar pigments such as copper. Identification of pigments is important as it directs cytologic interpretation, thus directly influencing patient diagnosis. This paper also presents basic iron metabolism, iron disorders in small animals, and laboratory assessment of iron disorders.

Important steps in bone marrow aspirate evaluation include determining if bone marrow evaluation is indicated; using appropriate aspirate collection, smear preparation, and staining techniques; and performing a systematic approach for the cytologic evaluation. The cytologic evaluation of bone marrow requires knowledge of the morphology of bone marrow cell types, the proportion of these cell types normally present, and the ability to evaluate overall cellularity of bone marrow. Accurate interpretation of bone marrow cytologic findings depends on evaluation of a current complete blood cell count. These components are the pillars of getting the most useful information in the diagnosis of hematologic disorders.

Cytology is commonly used to diagnose lymphoma and leukemia. Frequently, a diagnosis of lymphoproliferative disease can be obtained via cytology, and some of the common subtypes of canine lymphoma and leukemia can have characteristic cytologic features. Flow cytometry is a critical tool in the objective diagnosis and further characterization of lymphoma and leukemia. Features of the immunophenotype, such as expression of certain cell surface proteins or cell size, can provide important prognostic information. This review describes the cytologic features, flow cytometry immunophenotype, and immunophenotypic prognostic information for 6 major types of canine lymphoma and leukemia.

Cytology of bone is a useful diagnostic tool. Aspiration of lytic or proliferative lesions can assist with the diagnosis of inflammatory or neoplastic processes. Bacterial, fungal, and protozoal organisms can result in significant osteomyelitis, and these organisms can be identified on cytology. Neoplasms of bone including primary bone tumors such as osteosarcoma, chondrosarcoma, fibrosarcoma, synovial cell sarcoma, and histiocytic sarcoma and tumors of bone marrow including plasma cell neoplasia and lymphoma and metastatic neoplasia can result in significant bone lysis or proliferation and can be diagnosed effectively with cytology.

Fine-needle aspiration and cytologic examination should be a component of the diagnostic workup of skin masses. Cytologic examination may allow veterinarians to categorize neoplasms of the skin as epithelial, mesenchymal, or round cell and to determine the malignancy potential of the tumor. These results should provide veterinarians the ability to discuss with their clients the subsequent diagnostic considerations and appropriate treatment options for these tumors.

Synovial fluid analysis is a key component of the minimum database needed to diagnose and manage primary and secondary articular joint disorders. Unfortunately, preanalytical variables can drastically alter samples submitted for evaluation to veterinary laboratories and it is considered the stage at which most laboratory error occurs. This article addresses common sources of preanalytical variability and error that are seen in veterinary medicine. With consistent quality control and reporting of specimens, downstream clinical decision making and management of patients can be accelerated and improved.

Canine peritoneal fluid analysis results were retrospectively reviewed to assess the appropriateness of different classification schemes. Cutoffs of 3000 cells/μL and 2.5 g/dL protein are recommended. Analyzing the total nucleated cell count and total protein concentration is only the first step in peritoneal fluid analysis; microscopic examination, clinical presentation, and other laboratory data are all important in determining the final classification of peritoneal fluid analysis, keeping in mind that the most important aspect of fluid analysis is not what something is called, but whether it helps achieve a diagnosis. Discussion of effusion mechanisms, study observations, and recommended diagnostic steps after fluid analysis are included.

Linda M. Vap and Sarah B. Shropshire

Cytologic examination of the urine sediment in animals suspected of having urinary tract disease or lower urinary tract masses is one of the best means of distinguishing inflammation, infection, and neoplasia and can help determine if a positive dipstick result for hemoglobin/blood is due to hemorrhage or blood contamination. The quality of the specimen collection and handling plays an important role in the quality of results, the validity of interpretations, and selection of appropriate course of action. The method of sample collection aids localization of pathology. Air dry but do not heat fix, freeze, or expose films to formalin fumes, temperature extremes, or condensation.

Craig A. Thompson and Amy L. MacNeill

Cytology offers a rapid, relatively noninvasive means to identify lesions of all varieties including immune-mediated, degenerate, inflammatory, and neoplastic. One area that is particularly amenable to cytologic diagnosis is infectious disease. Organisms that can be seen and identified include fungal, bacterial, protozoal, parasitic, viral, and algal. Rapid identification of pathogenic organisms allows the practitioner to initiate treatment quickly, giving the patient the best chance for recovery.

VETERINARY CLINICS OF NORTH AMERICA: SMALL ANIMAL PRACTICE

RELATED INTEREST

Veterinary Clinics of North America: Exotic Animal Practice
January 2017, Volume 20, Issue 1
Exotic Animal Oncology
David Sanchez-Migallon Guzman, *Editor*

THE CLINICS ARE NOW AVAILABLE ONLINE!
Access your subscription at:
www.theclinics.com

Preface

Getting the Most from Your Cytology Samples

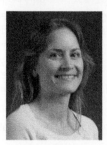

Amy L. MacNeill, DVM, PhD, DACVP
Editor

This issue of *Veterinary Clinics of North America: Small Animal Practice* is an eclectic grouping of articles that are focused on helping veterinarians optimize results they obtain from cytology samples. Articles include general information that is critical to collecting a good sample as well as pearls of wisdom about sample processing and interpretation that cannot be found in standard cytology texts.

Many of the topics in this issue discuss preanalytical considerations for sample collection and encourage readers to think about all the steps involved in cytologic evaluation of lesions. Topics that provide valuable sample processing information in addition to guiding the reader through sample interpretation include: "Preparation of Cytology Samples: Tricks of the Trade," "Bone Marrow Aspirate Evaluation," "Preanalytical Considerations for Joint Fluid Evaluation," and "Urine Cytology: Collection, Film Preparation, and Evaluation."

Other topics offer new information about the utility of cytology and advice about interpretation of cytology samples, including "Lymphoid Neoplasia—Correlations Between Morphology and Flow Cytometry" and "Analysis of Canine Peritoneal Fluid Analysis."

This issue also includes topics that are often overlooked in other publications, such as "Pigments: Iron and Friends" and "Cytology of Bone." These articles provide the reader with interesting and current information about cytologic findings and discuss how interpretation of the findings can be improved using special staining techniques.

Many topics in this issue include high-quality microscopic images that illustrate key points of the articles. Images found in "Cytology of Skin Neoplasms" and "Common Infectious Organisms" will be particularly beneficial to clinicians who use cytology in their practices.

We hope that the information provided in this issue of *Veterinary Clinics of North America: Small Animal Practice* is enjoyable to read and provides veterinarians with

Vet Clin Small Anim 47 (2017) ix–x
http://dx.doi.org/10.1016/j.cvsm.2016.09.001
0195-5616/17/© 2016 Published by Elsevier Inc.

vetsmall.theclinics.com

a valuable reference that helps them optimally use cytology to quickly and effectively diagnose diseases in their patients.

Amy L. MacNeill, DVM, PhD, DACVP
Clinical Pathology Section
Department of Microbiology, Immunology
and Pathology
College of Veterinary Medicine
and Biomedical Sciences
Colorado State University
Campus Delivery 1644
300 West Drake Road
Ft. Collins, CO 80523-1644, USA

E-mail address:
amy.macneill@colostate.edu

Preparation of Cytology Samples: Tricks of the Trade

A Russell Moore, DVM, MS

KEYWORDS

• Digital image • Cytology • Sample preparation • Romanowsky stain

KEY POINTS

• Cytology has many advantages; it is relatively quick, minimally invasive, and provides clinically useful results.
• To get ideal results, cytology does require some investment in time to acquire the skills to collect and evaluate the sample.
• Beyond reading and learning about how to perform these techniques, the next step is to practice and experiment with those techniques until the skills can be reliably used in the clinical setting.

TECHNIQUES FOR CYTOLOGIC PREPARATION

The quality of every cytologic evaluation is directly impacted by the quality of sample selection, collection, and preparation. Adherence to basic principles can significantly improve the usefulness of this simple and minimally invasive diagnostic test. Application of the principles covered in this article will help to improve the quality of cytologic preparations.

SAMPLE COLLECTION

Equipment

Minimal equipment is needed to collect and prepare cytologic samples. Additional information on staining and microscopic evaluation are discussed in following sections.

Needles

A 21- to 27-gauge needle is used for most settings. Generally, studies have found that needle size did not significantly affect cytologic adequacy, though admittedly, only needles ranging between 21 and 27 gauge were used.[1,2] Larger gauge needles may be helpful in poorly exfoliative sites, such as bone and suspected mesenchymal

The author has nothing to disclose.
Department of Microbiology, Immunology, and Pathology, College of Veterinary Medicine and Biomedical Sciences, Colorado State University, 311 Diagnostic Medical Center, 300 West Drake, Fort Collins, CO 80524, USA
E-mail address: ar.moore@colostate.edu

Vet Clin Small Anim 47 (2017) 1–16
http://dx.doi.org/10.1016/j.cvsm.2016.07.001

vetsmall.theclinics.com

tumors. Needle length depends on the depth of the lesion being evaluated; a 1- to 1.5-inch needle usually is sufficient.

Syringe

A 6-mL syringe will generally suffice for those techniques that require aspiration. Too large a syringe will apply too much pressor or be ungainly in the hand, whereas small syringes may not apply sufficient aspiration. A section of extension tubing between the needle and syringe can make collection easier.

Slides

Clean glass slides are imperative. Greasy or dirty slides prevent even distribution of the sample and introduce contaminants. Although these contaminations can usually be recognized as such by an experienced cytologists, they can also occasionally cause diagnostic confusion.

Location Selection

When deciding which area(s) to sample, start by considering the likely architecture of the lesion. There is typically an interface of normal host reactive or inflammatory cells surrounding many lesions. The center of fast-growing lesions often are composed of necrotic debris. Surfaces, especially ulcerated ones, often contain opportunistic bacteria, acellular crusts, and inflammation. Therefore, there are distinct advantages to aspirating multiple locations within a lesion.

Typically, sampling off the center of mass lesions are most rewarding diagnostically. Ulcerated lesions may need to be sampled deep to the ulcerated surface.[3] If multiple lesions are present, collection from both the older and newer lesions can demonstration the chronologic course of the pathology.

Site and Patient Preparation

One of the main advantages of cytology is the minimally invasive nature of sample collection. Minimally invasive does not mean that it is stress free to the patient. The patient should be restrained adequately; this may mean simple physical restraint for a compliant patient that is not undergoing a highly invasive technique. Painful procedures or anxious patients may benefit from analgesia and/or chemical restraint. If a sample is being collected from a lesion on the surface of the skin using the imprint/scraping technique, the surface should be sampled without clipping hair or cleaning the lesion. If a sample is being collected using fenestration or aspiration techniques, the area of interest can be cleaned (if necessary); however, hair does not need to be clipped.

Collection Techniques

Nonaspiration/fenestration collection

Nonaspiration collection has also been called fenestration or capillary collection. The lesion of interest is stabilized manually and the needle is advanced into the lesion and then withdrawn partly out of the lesion, redirected, and advanced again several times. This action will pack cells into the needle while causing a minimal amount of trauma. Multiple areas of the mass can thus be sampled at essentially the same time. One study in human thyroid tissue found that redirecting fewer than 4 times increased the nondiagnostic rate of subsequent samples.[4]

After redirecting the needle multiple times, the needle is removed from the lesion and connected to an air-filled syringe. The sample in the needle is then gently expelled onto a glass slide. A gentle hand is helpful when placing the aspirated material on the slide; insufficient pressure will leave sample in the needle. Overly aggressive expelling will splatter and disperse the material too much.

Nonaspiration techniques are ideal for lesions that exfoliate easily or have a high potential for hemorrhage.[1] They tend to be less useful in poorly exfoliative lesions.

Aspiration collection

The needle is connected to the syringe before sample collection for aspiration techniques. The lesion is stabilized manually and the needle advanced into the lesion. When the needle is in the desired location, the syringe plunger is pulled back and quickly released to create suction and collect cells while minimizing blood contamination. All suction should be relieved before withdrawing the needle from the tissue to keep from displacing the sample into the barrel of the syringe.

A portion of the sample will remain in the needle hub during collection. To use the sample in the needle hub fully, the syringe is removed from the needle, filled with air, and then used to expel the sample on a slide as described for the fenestration technique. If a portion of the sample is displaced into the syringe, the sample can be flushed out with a small amount of normal saline and handled as a fluid.

Aspiration techniques are most useful in solid lesions that need extra coercion during sampling, such as mesenchymal, fibrotic, or sclerosing lesions. They should not be used for samples that have a high propensity for hemorrhaging, both for the clinical aspect of excess hemorrhage in the patient and the deleterious effect that blood contamination has on cytologic diagnosis.[1]

Imprint/scraping

Imprint cytology samples can be gathered from accessible surfaces without an incision. The slide can be pressed onto ulcerated or upbraided surfaces. Alternately, the back edge of a blade or metal spatula can be used to scrape the surface and transfer material to a slide. If the intent is to evaluate the surface material, the site can be imprinted without cleaning. This type of collection can be advantageous in cases where the primary pathologic process is progressing from outside the epithelium inward, such as fungal, bacterial, and parasitic processes. If the goal to identify the underlying layer (such as a mass under an ulcerated area), cleaning the lesion of hemorrhage, exudation, or unwanted debris and hair may be appropriate. If this is not done, the sample will often consist only of surface crusts, necrotic debris, hemorrhage, or exuded inflammatory cells and normal bacterial flora. Often, collecting both the surface and deeper tissue is wise.

Tissue excision

Essentially any technique used for collection of histologic samples can be used to obtain cytologic samples. This includes Tru-Cut–type biopsies, bone marrow cores, wedge biopsies, or even small portions of endoscopically obtained pinch biopsies.[5–7] Studies generally find good agreement between concurrently collected cytologic and histologic specimens.[8]

It is imperative to realize that the appropriate time to collect cytologic samples from these types of tissue is before the sample is placed in formalin fixative. If cytologic samples are exposed to formalin fumes, the cells are damaged and the sample is nearly always nondiagnostic.

Brush cytology

There are a few locations that are only easily visualized endoscopically. These include the respiratory tract and upper and lower gastrointestinal tracts.[9] Cytologic samples can be collected using a cylindrical nylon brush passed over the surface several times then rolled onto the slide. Often, multiple collection attempts will be needed before an adequate sample is present on the slide.

FILM PREPARATION

The object of film preparation is to produce at least a few areas with a monolayer of cells that are intact and as close to their original orientation with each other as possible. At least a few areas with overly disrupted or overly thick areas are expected; samples composed only of dense or disrupted cells are not useful diagnostically.

Simply squirting sample onto a slide is typically insufficient, and some method of evenly distributing the material is required (**Fig. 1**). Many techniques for making films are described; each has their unique strengths and weaknesses. Every clinician does not need to be proficient in each of the below methods; however, mastery of at least a couple methods will provide an option of approaches.

Whichever technique is used, every slide should be labeled with a minimum of patient name or identification and the location of the sample. The tool used to label will depend on the slide and stain used. Even so-called "permanent" markers are often not permanent in some stain fixatives and solvents. A pencil is preferred if the slide is etched.

Squash Preparation

Despite the name, active squashing is not needed for a squash preparation (**Fig. 2**). A small amount of material is placed near 1 end of a slide. A second slide is lightly set on top of, and perpendicular to, the first slide. The 2 slides are then gently pulled apart.

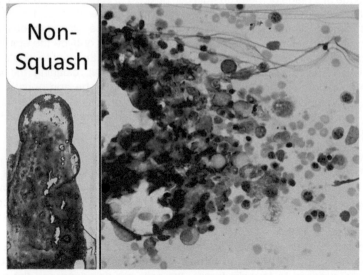

Fig. 1. Bone marrow sample from a dog. The same sample was prepared using multiple techniques (**Figs. 1–5**). A gross image of the slide (*left*) and photomicrograph of the best area for cytologic evaluation (*right*) is included. This sample was not smeared; an excess amount of sample was placed on the slide and then the slide was tilted to near vertical so that the fluid component would run off. Microscopically, the cells are trapped in dense areas of blood and tissue; few thin areas are present. A diagnosis could not be reached based on this sample. Stain: Wright-Giemsa; right panel, original magnification, ×500.

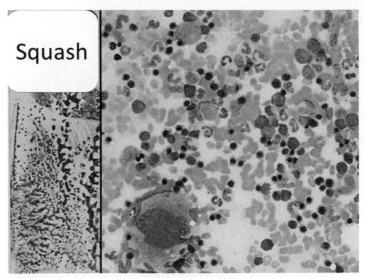

Fig. 2. Bone marrow sample from a dog. The same sample was prepared using multiple techniques (**Figs. 1–5**). A gross image of the slide (*left*) and photomicrograph of the best area for cytologic evaluation (*right*) is included. Squash preparation: a small amount of sample was placed on one slide and a second slide was laid over the first slide with minimal downward pressure. Both slides were pulled laterally apart. Most of this slide was of excellent diagnostic quality and allowed evaluation of the cells. Stain: Wright-Giemsa, right panel; original magnification, ×500.

With most samples, downward pressure is not needed; the weight of the second slide alone will spread the cells without rupturing them. If too much material is present on the slide, touching a third slide to the thick area will transfer some material, which can then be spread further.

Starfish Preparation

Starfish preparations have been described but cannot be recommended (**Fig. 3**). They are made by placing a small amount of material onto the slide and then using a needle, or other firm object, to drag the aspirated material out in multiple directions. The end result is an asterisklike spread of trailing edges around a central thick area. Much of the cellularity will be too thick for evaluation and the thin areas will typically contain predominantly ruptured cells.

Paintbrush Preparation

An acceptable variation of the starfish preparation involves using a soft-bristled artist's paint brush to spread the sample. This technique can be used to produce excellent quality slides. It does carry the risk of contamination from 1 sample to the next; meticulous cleaning of the spreading brush is required.

Pull Preparation

A pull preparation is essentially the same technique used to make a blood film (**Fig. 4**). A small droplet of material is placed on 1 end of a slide. A second slide is held at an acute angle (~30°) against the first slide and backed into the droplet. The sample is allowed to spread in the gap between the 2 slides and then the second slide is

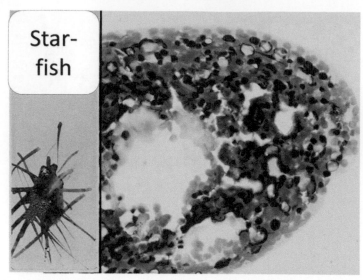

Fig. 3. Bone marrow sample from a dog. The same sample was prepared using multiple techniques (**Figs. 1–5**). A gross image of the slide (*left*) and photomicrograph of the best area for cytologic evaluation (*right*) is included. Starfish preparation: a needle was used to drag the sample outward from a centrally placed droplet. Notice in the gross image that most of the slide is very thick. The best areas for cytologic evaluation are confined to a small margin along the edge of the smear. Several areas in this slide consisted only of ruptured cells; this preparation was not diagnostically useful. Stain: Wright-Giemsa; right panel, original magnification, ×500.

smoothly advanced along the length of the first slide. The result should be a smear consisting of a body, monolayer, and feathered edge similar to a blood film. This technique works best with samples that have minimal to moderate amounts of fluid. It typically does not work well on samples that contain thick aggregates of cells or chunky or mucoid matrix that needs to be flattened before viewing.

Imprint Preparation

Imprints offer a quick primary evaluation of a sample collected for histopathology before biopsy samples are placed in formalin.[10] Most scraped or excised tissue will be covered in a layer of hemorrhage and interstitial fluid that will produce either hemodilute or poorly cellular samples if not removed. Before touching the sample to the slide, dab it on a gauze sponge or paper towel until the surface sticks slightly to the absorbent material. When the surface seems tacky, it is ready to make imprints on glass.

When making imprints, lateral movement across the surface should be minimized. Flat tissues that result from wedge excisions can be touched and lifted away from the slide. Round tissues from Tru-Cut biopsies or bone marrow cores should be rolled by lifting the lower edge on 1 side of the sample and moving the sample down the length of the slide (**Fig. 5**). Pushing across the top of the tissue produces a shearing force and ruptures most of the sample. It is also important to remember the original anatomic orientation of the sample. Imprinting the capsular surface of an abdominal organ will result in a slide of the mesothelial layer, whereas imprinting the cut surface will provide information on the parenchyma.

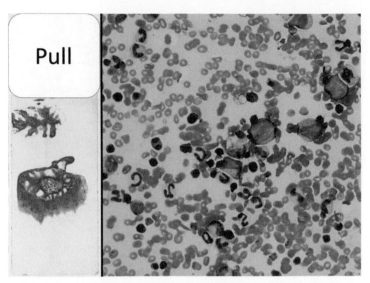

Fig. 4. Bone marrow sample from a dog. The same sample was prepared using multiple techniques (Figs. 1–5). A gross image of the slide (*left*) and photomicrograph of the best area for cytologic evaluation (*right*) is included. Pull preparation: a drop of sample was placed on 1 slide and a second slide was backed into the sample. After the material had spread between the 2 slides, the second slide was moved forward to pull the sample into a thinner layer. Useable areas of the slide are present. Although this technique is useful for many types of samples, it is usually not recommended for bone marrow preparations. Stain: Wright-Giemsa; right panel, original magnification ×500.

Fluid

Multiple types of fluid samples can be prepared for cytologic evaluation. This includes fluid from spaces that normally contain fluid (abdominal, thoracic, pericardial, synovial, and epidural spaces), pathologic accumulations of fluid (hematoma, edema, cyst, hygroma, etc), and diagnostic samples collected with the aid of fluid (flushes and washes). When fluids are handled appropriately, they are fairly stable; however, changes in the cellularity or growth of bacteria can occur in a relatively short period of time. Preparation of at least 1 or 2 slides within 1 hour of sample collection can help to minimize the effect of postcollection artifacts.[11] Preparation of fluid samples for cytology often entails some form of concentration of the cellularity. Several techniques are available.

Centrifuged sedimentation

Reference laboratories often use a specialized centrifuge (a cytocentrifuge), funnels, and filter paper to quickly prepare concentrated slides from fluid samples (**Fig. 6**). This equipment is relatively inexpensive and fairly easy to operate; however, alternate methods of fluid preparation can be used in the rare times that the typical veterinary clinic needs to handle a fluid sample in house. If sufficient volume of fluid is available, a traditional centrifuge and urine sedimentation protocol can be used. After the supernatant is removed, the sedimented material is resuspended and smeared on a slide.

Gravitational sedimentation

For samples with less available volume, a slightly more complex gravitational method can be accomplished with the help of some office supplies (**Fig. 7**).[12,13] This technique

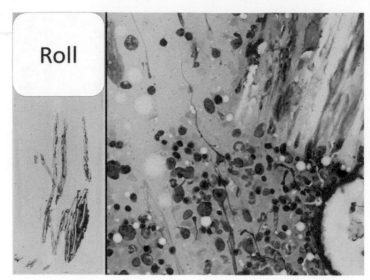

Fig. 5. Bone marrow sample from a dog. The same sample was prepared using multiple techniques (**Figs. 1–5**). A gross image of the slide (*left*) and photomicrograph of the best area for cytologic evaluation (*right*) is included. Roll preparation: a piece of the bone marrow core was rolled across the slide. Much of the sample was adequate. Notice where the cells are ruptured in the upper right corner of the microscopic image; shearing force was used instead of lifting to roll the sample over the surface. Stain: Wright-Giemsa; right panel, original magnification ×500.

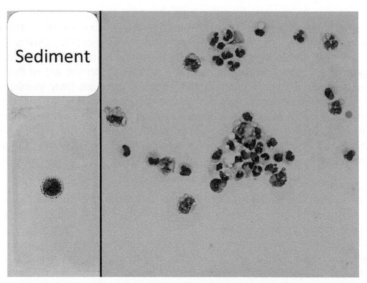

Fig. 6. Abdominal fluid from a dog with pancreatitis. Cytocentrifuge preparation: a cytocentrifuge was used to concentrate the cells in a small area of the slide while wicking away excess fluid. Note that the gross image (*left*) was made overly thick for photographic purposes. Individualized cells are apparent microscopically (*right*). Stain: Wright-Giemsa; right panel, original magnification ×500. Same case as **Fig. 8**.

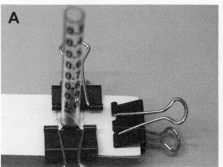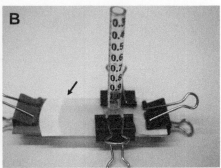

Fig. 7. A gravitational sedimentation system can be made with filter paper, a hole punch, a syringe, binder clips, and a glass slide. (*A*) Note that the hole in the filter paper is lined up underneath the barrel of the syringe. The binder clips keep the syringe, filter paper, and slide sandwiched together. (*B*) A fluid sample has been loaded into the syringe and allowed to stand. The cells in the sample will fall and adhere to the glass slide while the excess fluid will be wicked away (*arrow*). The resulting slide will look similar to what is produced by a cytocentrifuge (see **Fig. 6**).

involves sandwiching a piece of filter paper with a whole punched in it between a glass slide and the barrel of a 1-mL syringe that has had the hub cut off. Binder clips on the syringe finger flanges and slide are used to keep the contraption together. A relatively small volume of fluid, typically less than 0.25 mL, is loaded into the syringe barrel and allowed to stand for up to 30 minutes. Excess fluid will be wicked away into the filter paper and gravity will concentrate the cells into a small space on the slide.

This type of sedimentation chamber may produce slides with fewer cells and altered cell percentages when compared with paired cytocentrifuged samples, especially in samples with very low cell counts and low protein concentration.[13] Similar changes can be induced in cytocentrifuged samples by delaying sample preparation.[14] Perhaps the effects of the sedimentation chamber are owing to the significantly longer time involved in the protocol.

Line preparation

If only moderate cell concentration is needed, a line preparation can be used (**Fig. 8**). A line preparation is essentially a pull preparation that is ended before all of the fluid is smeared out. A small droplet of fluid is placed on one end of the slide. A second slide is held at an acute angle (~30°) to the first slide and backed in the droplet. When the fluid has sufficiently spread between the slides, the spreader slide is moved three-quarters of the way down the slide and then lifted directly up. The slide is then air dried and stained. The result should be a thin layer of fluid along much of the smear with a line of increased cellularity where the smear was terminated.

STAINING

Multiple stain protocols have been promulgated for cytology.[15,16] In veterinary cytology, Romanowsky stains are used routinely.

Romanowsky Stains

Romanowsky stain systems typically use an alcohol fixative and combination of dyes dissolved in either an aqueous or alcohol solution.[15,16] This family of stain was discovered after attempting to use moldy methylene blue stain; they provide good nuclear

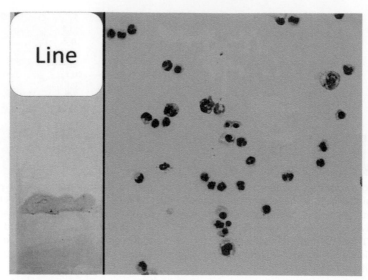

Fig. 8. Abdominal fluid from a dog with pancreatitis. Line preparation: a small amount of sample was placed at the frosted end of the slide. A second slide was backed into the sample, moved forward to approximately three-quarters of the length of the slide and then lifted straight up. A line of concentrated cellularity results (*gross image; left*). Cytologically, this results in cells that are slightly denser than a typical centrifuged sample; however, adequate cellular detail is present for a diagnosis (*right*). Stain: Wright-Giemsa; right panel, original magnification ×500. Same case as **Fig. 6.**

and cytoplasmic detail needed cytology and hematology.[16] For in-clinic laboratories, a quick Romanowsky stain such as Diff Quik (Siemens USA, Washington, DC) or similar stain is commonly used. They are ideal for in-clinic use because they are inexpensive and easy to use.

The technical details of stain development and function largely have little bearing on their actual use. However, several facets of stain preparation and use can be applied clinically.

- There are significant differences in stain concentration and dye composition between different Romanowsky stains. This results in varied tinctorial quality and differential staining between manufacturers and even batches of stain. Most cytologists have a familiar and favorite stain. If a sample is to be submitted to a diagnostic laboratory, submission of unstained slides that can be stained with a preferred stain is wise.
- Romanowsky stains typically include a chemical fixative designed to be used on air dried slides. Heat fixation (passing the slide over a flame or other heat source) is not needed and can destroy a beautifully collected and prepared slide.
- Slides that have been formalin fixed will not stain well with most Romanowsky stains. Even exposure to formalin fumes (as will happen when cytologic and histologic samples are packaged in the same box for shipping) can affect stain quality.
- Most stain solutions are saturated preparations of dye. Over time, the dye will precipitate out of solution, especially as solvent evaporates. For this reason, it is recommended to change, or at least filter, stains on a routine schedule. Many systems recommend changing stains weekly. If a slide has a considerable

amount of stain precipitate, a quick dip in the solvent (usually the first/fixative solution) will remove the precipitate (**Fig. 9**). Leaving the slide too long in the solvent can effectively destain the slide.

- Stain solutions will become exhausted with heavy use. When they are exhausted, they do not stain as effectively. Even if precipitation is not an issue, routinely changing the stain solutions is recommended.
- Stain cannot adequately penetrate thick areas of a preparation and can overstain thin areas; an adequately prepared slide is needed.
- Ideally, a properly stained slide will have good distinction of both cytoplasmic and nuclear detail (**Fig. 10**). It tends to be easier to understain than overstain a slide; however, both can occur.

Other Stains

Gram staining may be used on cytologic preparations to help characterize bacteria as gram positive or negative. Gram staining will also stain nonbacterial structures; therefore, using a gram stain to confirm the presence of bacteria is a questionable practice.

New methylene blue or other vital stains can occasionally be used for cytologic preparations if evaluation of a wet sample is needed.[17] These preparations provide only limited information compared with Romanowsky stains owing to lack of differential staining of cellular structures.

IN-HOUSE EVALUATION
Microscope Configuration

The configuration of a microscope for cytology or hematology is different than that used for unstained fluid samples, such as urine or fecal floatation preparations. For cytology, the condenser should be raised closer to the slide, the iris diaphragm opened, and there should be sufficient light to fully illuminate the sample of interest without producing shadows. A basic cytology microscope should have a low-power objective (usually ×5 or ×10), and 1 or 2 high-power objectives (×40, ×50, ×60, and/or ×100) to help evaluate finer details. Objectives with ×40 and ×60 magnification typically are dry lenses, whereas ×50 and ×100 objective lenses usually require emersion oil to focus on the sample.

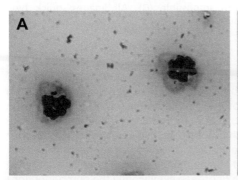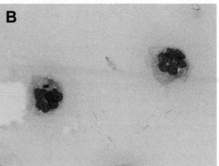

Fig. 9. The clinician had a suspicion of a septic abdomen when submitting this fluid. (*A*) There is an abundance of stain debris present, which can make identification of bacteria more challenging. However, the neutrophil on the left seems to have phagocytized bacteria. (*B*) Stain debris was removed with a quick dip in methanol and then the field was imaged again. The pair of cocci are much easier to see, whereas the particles of stain debris overlying the cytoplasm of the neutrophil on the right are now gone. Stain: Wright Giemsa; original magnification, ×1000.

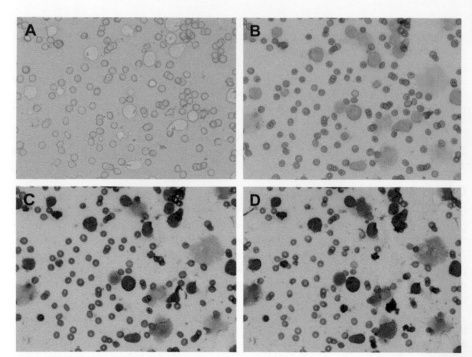

Fig. 10. A single field from a canine lymph node aspirate has been imaged as (*A*) unstained, (*B*) understained, (*C*) appropriately stained, and (*D*) overstained using a quick type manual Romanowsky stain. Determination of cellularity can be made on the unstained slide (*A*). Notice that both erythrocytes and larger nucleated cells are identifiable by their outline but, without staining, the cellular detail is not visible. There is poor cytologic distinction of cytoplasmic, nuclear, and nucleolar details in the understained image (*B*). Cytologic features are visible in *C*; most cells are larger than a neutrophil with minimal amounts of basophilic cytoplasm and a round to indented nucleus. As is typical for this type of stain, the nucleolar detail has been accentuated. This degree of staining is adequate to diagnose lymphoma. With overstaining, some of the finer nuclear and cytoplasmic details are lost, making interpretation more challenging but not impossible (*D*). All images: quick type Romanowsky stain; original magnification ×1000.

Evaluate for Sample Adequacy

Ideally, at least 1 slide from every case will be evaluated in-house for adequacy of preparation. This type of evaluation can be done quickly on low power and at the time of sample collection. The cells do not need to be identified but do need to be identifiable, meaning that cells are present, intact, and sufficiently thin to allow evaluation of cytoplasmic and nuclear detail. With practice, unstained slides can be used for this evaluation (see **Fig. 10**A). If the sample is deemed inadequate, resampling of the lesion can be performed before the patient leaves the premises. Studies have shown that evaluation at the time of collection can decrease significantly the number of non-diagnostic samples.[18]

Evaluate for a Diagnosis

A full evaluation of a slide starts with a scan of the complete slide at low power. The goals at this point are to note where the sample is and determine whether all parts of the slide have a similar population of cells. Next, a closer evaluation at a higher power can be performed to identify what is present. Although it is preferred to arrive at a definitive diagnosis in every case, this is not always possible. Placement of the sample into the broad categories of normal/hyperplastic, inflammation, or neoplasia can be clinically useful and often provides sufficient information to begin treatment. Subsequently, consultation with a more skilled pathologist or follow-up testing (including special staining or biopsy for histopathology) can be used to definitively diagnose the pathology definitively.

SUBMISSION TO A REFERENCE LABORATORY

Cytologic samples can be submitted to a reference laboratory for either a primary evaluation or consultation of challenging cases. Establishing a relationship with and consistently submitting to 1, or a few, cytologists may be helpful. Pathologists often provide a modifier to try to convey how confident they are in their interpretations. Data reveal a significant difference between pathologists in when they will use the same term and what degree of confidence they are trying to convey with a single term.[19,20] Similar differences occur in how clinicians interpret these modifiers.[21] Becoming familiar with how your routine cytologist writes can help you to gauge how to apply their results into the clinical interpretation of the case.

Multiple slides, including unstained slides, should be submitted. Considerable variability can occur between slides. If a slide was stained, evaluated in house, and felt to be diagnostic, it is wise to submit it for review. If questionable structures or cells are found during in-house evaluation, submission of a digital image of those structures may help communication with the pathologist.

History and Clinical Findings

Although cytologists are capable of arriving at conclusions without the history and clinical findings, they may be limited significantly by a lack of information. History and clinical findings often provide context for the significance of cytologic findings or help to narrow down differential lists. A good example of the usefulness of clinical findings is in the evaluation of neuroendocrine/naked-nuclei appearing tumors. These lesions are often indistinguishable from each other cytologically. Clinical data must be included to arrive at a diagnosis; a neuroendocrine appearing mass on the neck is likely to be a thyroid tumor, whereas similar cell morphology obtained from the perianal area is likely to be an apocrine gland adenocarcinoma.

Most referral laboratories have forms to help guide the clinician in communicating both what tests are desired and what types of history is required. Basic information with every submission should include signalment, a concise clinical history, a description of the lesion, and any other diagnostically relevant data. Submission of all 50 pages of the patient's record can be just as unhelpful as writing only "lump – please provide diagnosis."

Shipping

Cytology slides and fluid samples submitted to a reference laboratory must be packaged and shipped carefully. Slides and tubes that arrive in shards cannot provide a diagnostic sample, no matter how good the sample was before it was pulverized. Cardboard slide holders, although relatively inexpensive, often fail to keep slides intact. Polystyrene and firm plastic slide holders provide a more secure method of shipping.[22] Similarly, tubes should be packaged in a protective container (cardboard box or tube mailer) with the tubes tightly sealed.

Curriers and parcel handlers often have recommendations and policies for handling biologic samples and fluids. It is best to consult with the specific currier for their preferred methods. Generally, packaging should include an extra layer of a leak-proof container, sufficient absorbent material to prevent leakage should tubes break, and a sturdy external container.

In addition to preventing breakage, the sample should be protected from physical or chemical changes. Fluid samples in which cellularity will be examined should not be allowed to freeze or overheat. Air-dried slides are relatively temperature stable; however, cytologic specimens should be protected from exposure to formalin fumes and condensation or moisture.

DIGITAL IMAGE COLLECTION AND EVALUATION

Digital image–based telemedicine is becoming more common in both human and veterinary medicine. However, not all pathologists and reference laboratories are currently capable of or comfortable with interpreting still images from in-clinic slides. Some laboratories currently will provide an official report based on only submitted images; others will provide a provisional report contingent on review of the glass slide when it arrives in the laboratory, and others will comment informally but will not provide a report. Perhaps a good portion of the reason that pathologists are hesitant to review a small handful of still images lies in concerns over image quality and representativeness of the images.

Multiple systems are available for capturing digital images from a traditional microscope. These include large digital cameras specifically made for a microscope, traditional digital cameras, and smart phone cameras. All of these systems have been proven capable of taking adequate images.[23,24]

Adequate images can be taken by simply holding a camera close to a standard microscope's ocular lens.[25] A section of cardboard tubing (ie, paper towel or toilet paper roll) can be used to help stabilize the camera lens against the microscope and make lining up a shot easier. Several commercial adapters are available that can make capturing images using smart phones easier.[26]

Alternately, microscope attachments for smartphones have been developed.[27] Many of these systems are little more than a slide holder and light source; they rely on the smart phone lens and zoom for focus and magnification. These systems are designed as a replacement for a traditional microscope, not as a method of collecting images from a microscope. Their use in veterinary medicine has not yet been reported.

The technique used to capture an image will depend on the operator and the equipment being used. Basic criteria for a good digital image include the following:

- The sample being imaged should be of best possible quality. Excellent photography cannot overcome the effects of poorly stained slides, overly thick preparations, or insufficiently preserved cells.
- The structure(s) of interest should be centered in the field and as large as possible. This can be done using both the microscope's objectives and the zoom feature on the camera.
- The field should be illuminated adequately. The automatic white balancing and algorithms designed for image adjustment and compression on some phones can affect this.[28] Completely turning off image adjustments may be needed. Alternately, it may be helpful to establish white balance settings in an empty field and then use those settings in the desired field.

- The image should be in focus with adequate contrast. Note that automatic focus and image adjustments can affect this.[28] These features may need to be turned off.
- Multiple images (or video) should be taken, which provide a representation of multiple fields of view. Diagnosing based on 1 cell or 1 field is a very risky event and is not typically done even on glass slides. Demonstrating similar cells in multiple fields can help increase the confidence of a diagnosis.

SUMMARY

Cytology has many advantages; it is relatively quick, minimally invasive, and provides clinically useful results. Additionally, this technique requires minimal investment in equipment. To obtain ideal results, it does require some investment of time to acquire the skills to collect and evaluate the sample. Beyond reading and learning about how to perform these techniques, the next step is to practice and experiment with those techniques until the skills can be reliably used in the clinical setting.

REFERENCES

1. Leblanc CJ, Head LL, Fry MM. Comparison of aspiration and nonaspiration techniques for obtaining cytologic samples from the canine and feline spleen. Vet Clin Pathol 2009;38(2):242–6.
2. Cerit M, Yücel C, Göçün PU, et al. Ultrasound-guided thyroid nodule fine-needle biopsies–comparison of sample adequacy with different sampling techniques, different needle sizes, and with/without onsite cytological analysis. Endokrynol Pol 2015;66(4):295–300.
3. MacNeill AL. Cytology of canine and feline cutaneous and subcutaneous lesions and lymph nodes. Top Companion Anim Med 2011;26(2):62–76.
4. Zhu W, Michael CW. How important is on-site adequacy assessment for thyroid FNA? An evaluation of 883 cases. Diagn Cytopathol 2007;35(3):183–6.
5. Raskin RE, Messick JB, Raskin RE. Bone marrow cytologic and histologic biopsies: indications, technique, and evaluation. Vet Clin North Am Small Anim Pract 2012;42(1):23–42.
6. Powe JR, Canfield PJ, Martin PA. Evaluation of the cytologic diagnosis of canine prostatic disorders. Vet Clin Pathol 2004;33(3):150–4.
7. Mangelsdorf S, Teske E, v Bomhard W, et al. Cytology of endoscopically obtained biopsies for the diagnosis of chronic intestinal diseases in cats. Tierarztl Prax Ausg K Kleintiere Heimtiere 2015;43(1):15–20, 22.
8. Sharkey LC, Dial SM, Matz ME. Maximizing the diagnostic value of cytology in small animal practice. Vet Clin North Am Small Anim Pract 2007;37(2):351–72.
9. Caniatti M, da Cunha NP, Avallone G, et al. Diagnostic accuracy of brush cytology in canine chronic intranasal disease. Vet Clin Pathol 2012;41(1):133–40.
10. Clercx C, Wallon J, Gilbert S, et al. Imprint and brush cytology in the diagnosis of canine intranasal tumours. J Small Anim Pract 1996;37(9):423–7.
11. Bohn AA, Callan RJ. Cytology in food animal practice. Vet Clin North Am Food Anim Pract 2007;23(3):443–79, vi.
12. Mayhew IG, Beal CR. Techniques of analysis of cerebrospinal fluid. Vet Clin North Am Small Anim Pract 1980;10(1):155–76.
13. Wamsley HL. Clinical pathology. In: Platt SR, Olby NJ, editors. BSAVA manual of canine and feline neurology. 4th edition. Quedgeley (Gloucester): British Small Animal Veterinary Association; 2013. p. 36–58.

14. Fry MM, Vernau W, Kass PH, et al. Effects of time, initial composition, and stabilizing agents on the results of canine cerebrospinal fluid analysis. Vet Clin Pathol 2006;35(1):72–7.
15. Barcia JJ. The Giemsa stain: its history and applications. Int J Surg Pathol 2007; 15(3):292–6.
16. Dunning K, Safo AO. The ultimate Wright-Giemsa stain: 60 years in the making. Biotech Histochem 2011;86(2):69–75.
17. Hodges J. Using cytology to increase small animal practice revenue. Vet Clin North Am Small Anim Pract 2013;43(6):1385–408.
18. Nasuti JF, Gupta PK, Baloch ZW. Diagnostic value and cost-effectiveness of on-site evaluation of fine-needle aspiration specimens: review of 5,688 cases. Diagn Cytopathol 2002;27(1):1–4.
19. Christopher MM, Hotz CS. Cytologic diagnosis: expression of probability by clinical pathologists. Vet Clin Pathol 2004;33(2):84–95.
20. Lindley SW, Gillies EM, Hassell LA. Communicating diagnostic uncertainty in surgical pathology reports: disparities between sender and receiver. Pathol Res Pract 2014;210(10):628–33.
21. Christopher MM, Hotz CS, Shelly SM, et al. Interpretation by clinicians of probability expressions in cytology reports and effect on clinical decision-making. J Vet Intern Med 2010;24(3):496–503.
22. Meinkoth JH, Allison RW. Sample collection and handling: getting accurate results. Vet Clin North Am Small Anim Pract 2007;37(2):203–19.
23. Wimmer J, Dhurandhar B, Fairley T, et al. A novel smartphone-microscope camera adapter: an option for cytology consultation in low-resource environments. J Am Soc Cytopathol 2012;1(1):S124–5.
24. Lehman JS, Gibson LE. Smart teledermatopathology: a feasibility study of novel, high-value, portable, widely accessible and intuitive telepathology methods using handheld electronic devices. J Cutan Pathol 2013;40(5):513–8.
25. Bellina L, Missoni E. Mobile cell-phones (M-phones) in telemicroscopy: increasing connectivity of isolated laboratories. Diagn Pathol 2009;4:19.
26. Roy S, Pantanowitz L, Amin M, et al. Smartphone adapters for digital photomicrography. J Pathol Inform 2014;5(1):24.
27. Switz NA, D'Ambrosio MV, Fletcher DA. Low-cost mobile phone microscopy with a reversed mobile phone camera lens. PLoS One 2014;9(5):e95330.
28. Skandarajah A, Reber CD, Switz NA, et al. Quantitative imaging with a mobile phone microscope. PLoS One 2014;9(5):e96906.

Pigments: Iron and Friends

Lauren B. Radakovich, DVM, Christine S. Olver, DVM, PhD*

KEYWORDS

- Cytology • Prussian blue • Hemosiderin • Canine • Feline • Iron metabolism

KEY POINTS

- Serum iron is not a good indicator of total body iron stores.
- Serum ferritin correlates with total body iron stores, and when decreased, absolute iron deficiency can be diagnosed.
- Serum ferritin is an acute-phase protein and may not reflect iron stores when inflammation is present.
- Prussian blue stain highlights iron in cytology and histology samples.
- Special stains are required to differentiate pigment types definitively.

INTRODUCTION

Pigments are materials that change the color of either transmitted or reflected light due to absorption of specific wavelengths, and are commonly encountered in cytologic specimens. Cytologic analysis uses pigments by virtue of the Romanowsky staining process. Although various pigments exist in the natural world, they are more limited in cytologic samples because of the biochemical reactions involved in the staining process. The main components of these stains cause nucleic acids to appear blue to purple in color, while more alkaline cellular components take on a pink or eosinophilic color.[1] Common intracytoplasmic pigments are often various shades of blue, although these shades are often mixed with green, brown, yellow, and black. Therefore, there is much overlap in the appearance of many cellular pigments. As such, it is often difficult to distinguish pigments originating from different processes using the microscopic appearance of cytologic samples. Differentiation is important, as it can affect overall interpretation of the sample and may influence final diagnosis and treatment plans for the patient. The aim of this article is to introduce a broad spectrum of pigments commonly encountered in cytologic samples. The authors place a special emphasis on iron, as this is among the most common pigments observed.

The authors have nothing to disclose.
Department of Microbiology, Immunology, and Pathology, College of Veterinary Medicine and Biomedical Sciences, Colorado State University, 1644 Campus Delivery, Fort Collins, CO 80523, USA
* Corresponding author.
E-mail address: Christine.Olver@ColoState.edu

Vet Clin Small Anim 47 (2017) 17–29
http://dx.doi.org/10.1016/j.cvsm.2016.07.002
vetsmall.theclinics.com

Additionally, because iron is such an important biometal with a complicated homeo-static system, the article begins with an overview of mammalian iron metabolism, and then moves on to cytologic appearance of iron and other pigments.

MAMMALIAN IRON METABOLISM
Functions of Iron

Iron is an element essential for life and maintaining normal organism function. In mammals, the vast majority of iron is used to synthesize hemoglobin, the oxygen-carrying protein in erythrocytes. It is also necessary for the production of myoglobin, oxidative phosphorylation within mitochondria, DNA synthesis, and making iron–sulfur-containing proteins.[2] While iron is critical for survival and its deficiency can lead to anemia, it is also dangerous in high amounts, as it can promote free radical damage. It plays a central role in the Fenton reaction, in which oxidation reduction (redox) reactions with hydrogen peroxide release hydroxyl and hydroperoxyl radicals.[3,4] These reactive oxygen species (ROS) promote lipid peroxidation and DNA damage.

Iron Absorption

Because iron is necessary for life but is also toxic in excess, mammals have developed an intricate system for its regulation and availability. Surprisingly, mammals have no designated mechanism for iron excretion. Rather, total body iron is regulated by controlling how much is absorbed through the gastrointestinal (GI) tract. Iron can be absorbed in either heme (from animal sources) or non-heme (from plant sources) forms. Each form is transported across the enterocyte's apical membrane by a transport protein. Once within the enterocyte cytoplasm, iron may be stored within ferritin, a cytosolic protein that can bind thousands of Fe^{3+} particles, thus maintaining iron in a soluble and nontoxic form. If the body is iron replete, iron will remain within enterocytes as ferritin and be lost with normal sloughing of the GI tract epithelial surface. If there is a need for iron, as with iron deficiency or anemia, the ingested iron will be transported through the basolateral side of the enterocyte via ferroportin, the only cellular iron exporter identified to date.[5] After passing through ferroportin, iron is oxidized to the ferric form by hephaestin, a ferroxidase on the basolateral enterocyte membrane, to mediate binding of iron to the plasma protein transferrin.

Iron Transport, Uptake, and Recycling

Transferrin is the transport protein that carries iron throughout the bloodstream to reach its targets, primarily the erythroid cells of the bone marrow. Each unit of transferrin can carry 2 molecules of ferric (Fe^{3+}) iron.[6] Iron must be bound to transferrin within the blood to prevent oxidant damage. Once iron-bound transferrin reaches the bone marrow, it binds to rubriblasts (the earliest erythrocyte precursors) via the transferrin receptor (TfR1). The resulting complex is internalized within an endosome, ultimately resulting in the release of iron from transferrin. Iron exits the endosome while the empty transferrin receptor is recycled to the exterior of the cell, where it can then bind more iron, if needed.[7]

Macrophages within the splenic red pulp also play a major role in regulating iron availability. Most of the iron arriving at the bone marrow is recycled from these macrophages. As erythrocytes become senescent, they are cleared from the blood via erythrophagocytosis by macrophages (**Fig. 1**). Macrophages also have receptors CD163 and CD91 to scavenge iron from haptoglobin-bound hemoglobin and hemopexin-bound heme, respectively. Macrophages can also endocytose transferrin-bound iron via TfR1 (CD71). Once senescent red blood cells, heme, and hemoglobin

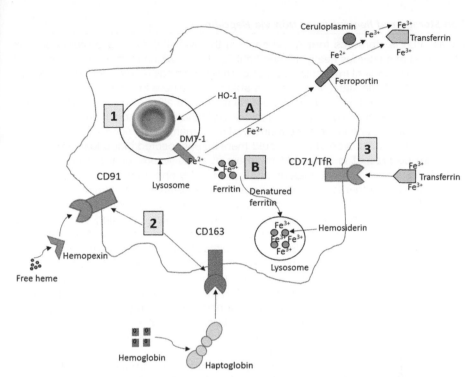

Fig. 1. Macrophage handling of iron. Intracellular iron is derived from multiple sources. 1. Senescent erythrocytes are cleared from the blood via erythrophagocytosis. 2. Macrophages also have receptors CD163 and CD91 to scavenge iron from haptoglobin-bound hemoglobin and hemopexin-bound heme, respectively. 3. Macrophages can also endocytose transferrin-bound iron via TfR1 (CD71). Once senescent red blood cells, heme, and hemoglobin are endocytosed, heme is degraded by heme-oxygenase 1 (HO-1) to release iron (and biliverdin), which is then exported from the endosome via DMT1. Likewise, when transferrin-bound iron binds to TfR, the complex is internalized; acidification of the endosome results in the reduction of iron, promoting its release from transferrin. The ferrous iron exits the endosome via DMT1, while TfR is returned to the cell membrane. Once iron is present in macrophages, it has 2 potential fates: (A) it can be exported through ferroportin, where it is oxidized by ceruloplasmin so it can bind transferrin, or (B) iron can be stored in the macrophage's cytoplasm in ferritin. Should ferritin stores become maximally filled, then hemosiderin begins to accumulate in the lysosome.

are endocytosed, heme is degraded by heme-oxygenase 1 (HO-1) to release iron (and biliverdin), which is then exported from the endosome via DMT1. Likewise, when transferrin-bound iron binds to TfR, the complex is internalized; acidification of the endosome results in the reduction of iron, promoting its release from transferrin. The ferrous iron exits the endosome via DMT1, while TfR is returned to the cell membrane.[8] Once iron is present in macrophages, it has 2 potential fates:

1. It can be exported through ferroportin, where it is oxidized by ceruloplasmin (a ferroxidase similar to hephaestin) to then bind transferrin.
2. Iron can be stored in the macrophage's cytoplasm in ferritin. Should ferritin stores become maximally filled, then hemosiderin begins to accumulate, as will be described.

Iron Storage and Regulation of Iron via Hepcidin

Excess iron is stored as ferritin, primarily in the liver. Ferritin is a protein complex comprised of numerous heavy (H) and light (L) chains, which form a protective shield around iron to prevent free radical damage. The H chain has ferroxidase activity, keeping iron in the ferric state, which is less able to participate in the deleterious Fenton reaction. The L chain is involved in electron transfer to allow iron release from ferritin when there is peripheral demand.[9] Iron stores, in the form of hemosiderin, are also present in the spleen and in the bone marrow of most mammalian species. These stores serve as a backup source of iron should there be unexpected blood loss. Iron stores may also be present in increased numbers in areas where local hemorrhage has occurred, such as in hematomas or within the local lymph node near an injured site. Hemosiderin is another storage form of iron that is a complex of ferritin and denatured ferritin. It is a nonsoluble form of iron that forms when there is iron overload. Essentially, ferritin becomes oversaturated with iron molecules, resulting in damage to ferritin. This damage allows iron to come into contact with redox reactive molecules in the cell cytoplasm, initiating free radical damage. The cell's response to this free radical damage is autophagy, where the damaged ferritin is engulfed by lysosomes. Damaged and degraded ferritin within lysosomes is classified as hemosiderin.[10] Cats lack stainable iron in bone marrow for unknown reasons; however, iron may be noted in marrow of cats with intravascular hemolysis and myeloproliferative disorders.[11,12] The body relies on iron stores to support hemoglobin synthesis when iron becomes scarce, as seen with an iron-poor diet (uncommon in dogs and cats on commercial diets) or chronic external blood loss.

When iron stores reach a maximum level and further absorption carries the risk of ROS formation, the liver is stimulated to produce hepcidin, the master iron regulator.[13] Hepcidin, encoded by the *Hamp* gene, is a peptide secreted by the liver in response to high total body iron levels. Hepcidin binds to ferroportin, resulting in its internalization and degradation. Subsequently, ingested iron cannot be exported from enterocytes; thus no iron is absorbed into the bloodstream. Likewise, iron cannot be exported from macrophages or hepatocytes. The result is a decreased amount of iron present in the bloodstream available to bone marrow erythroblasts.

Hepcidin is also induced by systemic inflammation, primarily through interleukin-6 (IL-6) activation. IL-6 induced production of hepcidin is an attempt by the body to sequester iron from potential invading pathogens. If inflammation is chronic, *functional* iron deficiency often develops. This term refers to ongoing iron sequestration within macrophages and duodenal enterocytes, thus limiting iron bioavailability to the bone marrow. Eventually, this iron sequestration can lead to anemia. This inflammation-induced anemia is termed anemia of chronic disease (ACD) or anemia of inflammation. Hepcidin production is inhibited when iron deficiency, tissue hypoxia, and anemia are present.[14] In the absence of hepcidin, ferroportin remains on enterocyte, hepatocyte, and macrophage membranes, thus allowing iron to be readily absorbed and cycled throughout the body.

LABORATORY ASSESSMENT OF IRON STATUS

Many tests are available for veterinarians to assess iron status in their patients. When there is concern about iron status, it is generally recommended to run a panel of tests, as this provides more useful information than any single test, alone. **Table 1** outlines the most common tests for iron status and the expected results for absolute and functional iron deficiency. Veterinarians typically first notice a potential problem in iron status by examining variables on a routine complete blood cell (CBC) count. The mean

Table 1
Expected results in absolute and functional iron deficiency

	HCT	MCV	SeFe	TIBC	% Sat	CHr	Ferritin	Marrow Stores
Absolute Iron Deficiency	N - Dec	Dec	Dec	Inc	Dec	Dec	Dec	Dec
Functional Iron Deficiency	N - Dec	N - Dec	Dec	Dec	N	N - Dec	N - Inc	N - Inc

Abbreviations: % sat, percent transferrin saturation; CHr, reticulocyte hemoglobin content; Dec, decreased; HCT, hematocrit; Inc, increased; MCV, mean cell volume; N, normal; SeFe, serum iron; TIBC, total iron binding capacity.

cell volume (MCV) is often decreased when iron deficiency is present. Unfortunately, this is not a sensitive test, and the MCV will decrease only when there are enough microcytic erythrocytes present to move the MCV below the reference interval, which can take weeks to months.[15] If available, examination of erythrocyte volume histograms may reveal a population of emerging microcytes, even if the MCV is still within the reference interval. Microcytosis may also be present with chronic inflammation caused by iron sequestration in macrophages resulting in functional iron deficiency.[16] Mean cell hemoglobin concentration (MCHC) is also typically decreased in iron deficiency. If absolute or functional iron deficiency goes on long enough, anemia will eventually develop.

Recently, there has been much interest in how reticulocyte indices may enhance the understanding of iron status, particularly in identifying early iron deficiency. Because reticulocytes reflect the marrow iron status from the past 3 to 5 days, their iron content may be more useful than the iron content of mature erythrocytes.[17,18] Reticulocyte hemoglobin content (CHr) has garnered the most attention of the reticulocyte indices. In the absence of inflammatory disease, CHr decreases with iron deficiency before changes would be noted in erythrocyte MCV or MCHC, as demonstrated in an experimental model of nutritional iron deficiency,[19] as well as in blood donor dogs.[20] Unfortunately, studies have revealed that reticulocyte indices, including CHr, are unable to differentiate absolute from functional iron deficiency. CHr is decreased in both absolute and functional iron deficiency secondary to inflammatory disease in dogs.[21–23]

In addition to hematologic variables available on CBC, there are also serum tests of iron status. These include serum iron, total iron binding capacity (TIBC), percent transferrin saturation (%sat), and serum ferritin. Serum iron is a measure of how much iron is present bound to transferrin. It is increased with hemolysis, iron supplementation, transfusions, and administration of glucocorticoids in dogs.[15] Serum iron is decreased with iron deficiency, inflammation (due to functional iron deficiency), hypothyroidism, and renal disease. It can also vary diurnally.[24] Because it is affected by so many variables, serum iron is not a specific test to assess patient iron status. Total iron binding capacity is essentially a measure of how much transferrin is present. It is increased when there is absolute iron deficiency and decreased when there is inflammation, since transferrin is a negative acute phase protein. Percent saturation of transferrin is typically less than 20% when absolute iron deficiency is present.[25] Serum ferritin reflects total iron stores, and when decreased, absolute iron deficiency can be diagnosed. Serum ferritin is increased with inflammation (ferritin is a positive acute phase protein), hemolysis, liver injury (liver is major source of ferritin), and some neoplasias.[15,26] Serum ferritin assays for dogs and cats are available through Kansas State University.

Although invasive, bone marrow assessment of iron stores is the current gold standard to evaluate for iron deficiency in dogs. Prussian blue staining is performed on aspirate smears and/or core biopsy samples to highlight iron (Prussian blue stain will be discussed in more detail). With absolute iron deficiency, iron stores will be markedly decreased to absent. With functional iron deficiency, they will be normal to increased because of sequestration within macrophages.

MAJOR IRON DISORDERS SEEN IN VETERINARY MEDICINE
Iron Deficiency

Iron deficiency is more commonly recognized than iron overload disorders. For more in-depth discussion of iron disorders, readers are directed to a recent review.[25] Please refer to **Table 2** for a brief overview of major iron disorders seen in veterinary medicine. Absolute iron deficiency in small animal patients is typically due to chronic, external blood loss. Nutritional iron deficiency is rare when commercial diets are fed. The most common sources of external blood loss include severe ectoparasitism in kittens and puppies and GI bleeding in adult animals. GI bleeding may result from upper GI ulceration secondary to nonsteroidal anti-inflammatory drug (NSAID) use, ulcerated GI mass lesions, and GI parasitism.

As mentioned previously, animals can also suffer from functional iron deficiency in the presence of chronic inflammation caused by the ferroportin-degrading action of hepcidin. Chronic inflammation can result in functional iron deficiency and eventually anemia of chronic disease, if unresolved. Conditions that often include ACD include neoplasia, immune-mediated disorders, endocrinopathies, chronic kidney disease, and ongoing infections, among others. To complicate matters further, both absolute and functional iron deficiency can exist simultaneously. This combinatorial iron deficiency may occur in patients with a chronic disease, such as cancer, who are also receiving NSAID medications that may cause gastric ulceration and bleeding. At this time, there are no laboratory tests that can accurately identify these patients, as ferritin is unreliable in the face of inflammation. Identification of absolute iron deficiency, even when inflammation is present, is important, because these animals benefit from iron supplementation.

Iron Overload

Iron overload disorders are less common than iron deficiency in companion animals. Excess iron is detrimental to cellular function due it its potential to induce free radicals,

---

Table 2
Major iron disorders seen in veterinary medicine

Iron Deficiency Disorders	Iron Overload Disorders

Absolute iron deficiency
  Chronic external blood loss
  • Blood-sucking parasites
  • GI ulceration (NSAID-related, ulcerated neoplastic lesion)
  • Ongoing blood donation
  Iron-poor diet
Functional iron deficiency
  Inflammatory disorders
Miscellaneous disorders with suspect iron derangement
  • Portosystemic shunts
  • Breed associated microcytosis
	Hemochromatosis (usually secondary in animals)
	  • Repeat blood transfusions
	  • Pyruvate kinase deficiency
	Hemosiderosis
	Ongoing hemolysis
	Oversupplementation with iron
	Chronic inflammation (local iron sequestration in macrophages can cause local free radical damage)

which damage DNA, lipids, and proteins within the cell. This free radical damage not only harms the cell but also incites the inflammatory process. In people, hereditary hemochromatosis is a disorder resulting in lack of functional hepcidin activity. As a result, iron is continuously absorbed from the GI tract, resulting in total body iron overload.[27] Although hereditary hemochromatosis has not been described in dogs or cats, hemochromatosis secondary to repeated blood transfusions[28] and due to erythrocyte pyruvate kinase deficiency in dogs and cats resulting in chronic hemolysis[29] is recognized.

HOW TO DETECT IRON CYTOLOGICALLY

Iron is commonly encountered in cytologic specimens, particularly in the form of hemosiderin. With Wright Giemsa stain, iron is typically green to dark blue in color and is present in globules of varying size. The color of hemosiderin is variable, however, and may be yellow, gold, light green, light or dark blue, and black (**Fig. 2**). It is most commonly seen within the cytoplasm of macrophages, especially from sites where there has been recent or ongoing hemorrhage (**Figs. 3** and **4**). Hemosiderin may be seen free within the background as well (see **Fig. 2**). Several other noniron pigments have a similar cytologic appearance. Cytologic clues may help differentiate whether a pigment is iron. In cases of hemorrhage, there may be an abundance of intact erythrocytes within the background. Phagocytosis of intact erythrocytes may be noted in macrophages along with hemosiderin (see **Fig. 3**). However, these context clues may not always be present to help determine the nature of blue globular pigment. Fortunately, Prussian blue staining is a readily available staining procedure that is specific for iron.

Prussian blue is a histochemical stain, although it is successfully applied to cytologic specimens. It is a very sensitive assay, able to detect very small quantities of iron. The procedure is simple and consists of adding hydrochloric acid to either an unstained or previously stained slide to denature proteins binding iron. Then a solution of potassium ferrocyanide is added, which binds to ferric iron molecules, resulting in an

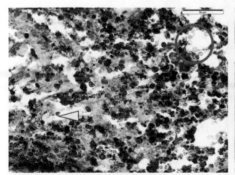 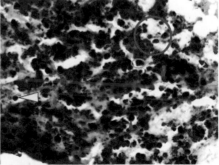

Fig. 2. This cytologic specimen comes from a lymph node aspirate containing previous hemorrhage. The hemosiderin granules are cell-free. The specimen on the left is stained with Wright Giemsa, and shows that hemosiderin ranges from a golden–yellow (*red circle*) to golden–brown (*red arrowhead*) to green (*yellow arrowhead*) to black (*green circle*). The image on the right is stained with Prussian blue to show iron-containing granules, and is the same field as that shown in the left-sided image. The shapes outlining or pointing to blue staining granules exactly match those in the left-sided image. These figures show that regardless of the Wright Giemsa appearance of hemosiderin, it will stain positively for iron.

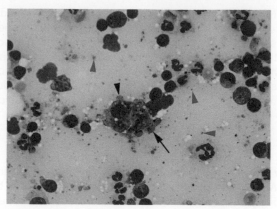

Fig. 3. Eythrophagocytic macrophage with hemosiderin. This sample is derived from a lymph node with suppurative inflammation and hemorrhage. The macrophage in the center of the image contains erythrocytes (*black arrow*), and hemosiderin (*black arrowhead*) presenting as yellow, green, blue, and black granules of variable size. There is also free hemosiderin in the background (*red arrowheads*).

insoluble blue pigment. A red counterstain is then used to visualize other cellular elements such as nuclei and cytoplasm. The iron present is visualized as the bright blue pigment.

Hematoidin is a golden yellow, refractile crystalline pigment that results from erythrocyte breakdown. Although it does not contain iron, it is often present within lesions that contain abundant erythrophagocytosis and resulting hemosiderin (see **Fig. 4**). Hematoidin is a breakdown product of the heme molecule after the iron has been transferred to apoferritin. The porphyrin ring opens to produce biliverdin, and under

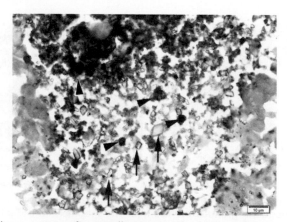

Fig. 4. This sample represents a fine needle aspirate of a subcutaneous hemorrhage. There is an accumulation of erythrocyte breakdown products including hemosiderin (*arrowheads*), which ranges from green to blue to black globular pigment and hematoidin (*arrows*). Hematoidin is a golden, typically rhomboid shaped, erythrocyte breakdown product that does not contain iron. Rather, hemoglobin is broken down into crystallized bilirubin when the environment is hypoxic. Erythrocytes are seen aggregated on the periphery of the image.

conditions of low oxygen tension, biliverdin is reduced to crystalline hematoidin. Typically hematoidin is rhomboid in shape, but it can also exist as needle-like crystals.

PIGMENTS THAT MASQUERADE AS IRON

As mentioned previously, other pigments may appear green or blue in color and can be confused with hemosiderin. These will be described.

Melanin

Melanin is a brownish-black pigment typically found in cells within the basal epithelial layer in pigmented animals. It can be seen in a variety of cytologic specimens including melanomas, tumors of the basal layer of the epidermis, and in lymph nodes draining heavily pigmented areas (**Fig. 5A**). Melanin granules in epithelial cells are uniform, rod-shaped, and are typically green, brown, or yellow in color. In melanocytes, including those of melanomas, granules are uniform, bright green, small, and round to rod-shaped.

Melanophages

When there is an abundance of melanin, macrophages often phagocytize it, and it is noted cytologically as globular green to brownish-black material within the cytoplasm (**Fig. 5B**). These melanin-laden macrophages, or melanophages, can be distinguished from melanocytes by the globular nature of the cytoplasmic melanin due to the melanin being packaged into lysosomes. Melanomacrophages are difficult to distinguish from hemosiderin-laden macrophages. Melanin does not stain positively with Prussian blue, so Prussian blue staining is one of the best ways to distinguish globular melanin from hemosiderin in cytologic samples.

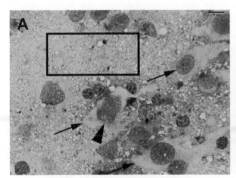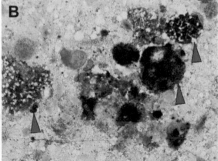

Fig. 5. This cytology is prepared from a fine needle aspirate of a mandibular lymph node that is draining an oral malignant melanoma. Melanin stains green with Wright Giemsa stain and can be difficult to differentiate from hemosiderin without applying additional staining techniques. Panel A shows several elongated melanocytes with a variable amount of green pigment (*arrows*). The arrowhead is pointing to the finely granular green pigment that is typical of melanin in melanocytes. The box highlights free melanin in the background. Panel B shows numerous melanophages, 3 of which are noted with the red arrowheads. Melanin in melanophages is typically more globular than that in melanocytes, and the melanophages are round (not elongated), with abundant pigment-containing cytoplasm, and single small nuclei. Melanin does not stain blue with Perl's Prussian blue stain.

Lipofuscin

Lipofuscin is an aging wear-and-tear pigment that accumulates in many cell types. Lipofuscin and lipofuscin-like pigments are insoluble aggregates of oxidized and indigestible proteins, along with carbohydrates, lipids, and incorporated transition metals (eg, iron and copper).[30] They appear green to green–blue to blue in cytologic specimens that have been stained with standard cytologic stains, and they can be confused with hemosiderin in macrophages and bile in hepatocytes. In cytology, lipofuscin is most commonly noted within liver samples. The amount of lipofuscin present in cells is directly proportional to the age of the cell, since the damaged and insoluble proteins cannot be digested. Lipofuscin does not stain positively with Prussian blue unless there is significant iron associated with the granules. Lipofuscin pigment can be specifically stained with Sudan black B (a lipophilic stain), glypican-3, Luxol fast blue, periodic acid Schiff, and acid-fast procedures.[31] Additionally, lipofuscin autofluoresces when excited at 360 nm.[30]

Copper

Copper is another pigment typically noted within hepatocytes. It is a pale but bright green and somewhat refractile (**Fig. 6**). Copper in hepatocytes is associated with lipofuscin. The presence of copper can be confirmed using rhodamine or rubeanic acid.

Phagocytized Material

Macrophages often contain material that is indistinguishable in cytologic appearance from hemosiderin. These pigments may originate from leukocytophagy or phagocytosis of secretory product or cystic material. When macrophages phagocytize leukocytes, the digested nuclear DNA may appear as a homogeneous blue material. Often the origin of that material as cellular DNA can be surmised by finding other macrophages in the sample that have more obvious intracytoplasmic phagocytized leukocytes. Other material that may masquerade as hemosiderin includes keratin (from phagocytosis of keratin in inflamed keratin-containing lesions), secretory product from mammary tumors, or other cystic lesions (**Fig. 7**). These pigments do not contain iron, and thus do not stain with Prussian blue.

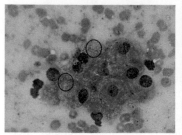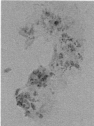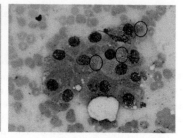

Fig. 6. Green pigment caused by copper accumulation in hepatocytes. The Wright Giemsa stained hepatocytes seen on the left and right show a refractile light green granular material in the cytoplasm. Several of the aggregates are circled, but the pigment is broadly dispersed within the hepatocyte cytoplasm. The center image shows hepatocytes from the same sample stained with rhodamine stain, which reacts with the copper to produce an orange pigment.

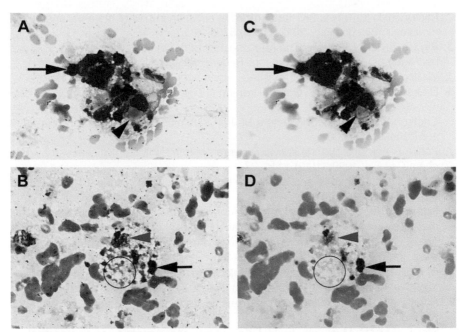

Fig. 7. Not all intracytoplasmic blue pigment is iron. A–D are from images from a cytology collected by fine needle aspirate from a cystic perianal gland tumor. There were abundant macrophages containing intracytoplasmic light to dark blue pigment. A and B are Wright Giemsa stained, while C and D are the same cells stained with Perl's Prussian blue to detect iron. Each shape or arrow is highlighting the same structure in both Wright Giemsa stained and Perl's Prussian blue stained samples. The black arrows point to classic dark blue/black pigment that stains positively for iron in the Perl's Prussian blue Stain. The black arrowhead points to blue material that stains pink, or iron negative, on the Perl's Prussian blue stain, indicating that it is not iron, and more likely phagocytosed cystic material (probably keratin). The red arrowhead points to the nucleus of the macrophage in B and D, and the black circle outlines a pale blue pigment that also does not stain with Perl's Prussion blue stain.

SUMMARY

Iron is commonly detected in cytologic specimens, and it can be differentiated from similar-appearing pigments by positive staining with Perl's Prussian blue. There are guidelines for deciphering what is iron/hemosiderin and what is not, and significance of other pigments:

- If there is evidence of erythrophagocytosis, then pigment is likely hemosiderin.
- Where melanoma is suspected, Prussian blue should be performed to rule out iron.
- If there is evidence of secretory product or keratin, then phagocytized cystic material should be suspected.
- Defining what is iron and what is not is important in the following cases:
  - Detection of previous hemorrhage in bronchoalveolar lavage samples.
  - Differentiating melanin/melanophages from hemosiderin/hemosiderophages.

REFERENCES

1. Houwen B. Blood film preparation and staining procedures. Clin Lab Med 2002; 22(1):1–14.

2. Pantopoulos K, Porwal SK, Tartakoff A, et al. Mechanisms of mammalian iron homeostasis. Biochemistry 2012;51(29):5705–24.
3. Rigg T, Taylor W, Weiss J. The rate constant of the bimolecular reaction between hydrogen peroxide and ferrous ion. Experientia 1954;10(5):202–3.
4. Walling C. Fenton's reagent revisited. Acc Chem Res 1975;8(4):125–31.
5. Drakesmith H, Nemeth E, Ganz T. Ironing out Ferroportin. Cell Metab 2015;22(5): 777–87.
6. Crichton RR, Charloteaux-Wauters M. Iron transport and storage. Eur J Biochem 1987;164(3):485–506.
7. Ponka P, Lok CN. The transferrin receptor: role in health and disease. Int J Biochem Cell Biol 1999;31(10):1111–37.
8. Ganz T. Macrophages and systemic iron homeostasis. J Innate Immun 2012; 4(5–6):446–53.
9. Finazzi D, Arosio P. Biology of ferritin in mammals: an update on iron storage, oxidative damage and neurodegeneration. Arch Toxicol 2014;88(10):1787–802.
10. Theil EC. Ferritin: the protein nanocage and iron biomineral in health and in disease. Inorg Chem 2013;52(21):12223–33.
11. Blue JT. Myelofibrosis in cats with myelodysplastic syndrome and acute myelogenous leukemia. Vet Pathol 1988;25(2):154–60.
12. Harvey JW. Myeloproliferative disorders in dogs and cats. Vet Clin North Am Small Anim Pract 1981;11(2):349–81.
13. Steinbicker AU, Muckenthaler MU. Out of balance–systemic iron homeostasis in iron-related disorders. Nutrients 2013;5(8):3034–61.
14. Grimes CN, Giori L, Fry MM. Role of hepcidin in iron metabolism and potential clinical applications. Vet Clin North Am Small Anim Pract 2012;42(1):85–96.
15. Harvey J. Iron metabolism and its disorders. In: Kaneko J, Harvey J, Bruss M, editors. Clinical biochemistry of domestic animals. 6th edition. San Diego (CA): Academic Press; 2008. p. 259–85.
16. Gavazza A, Rispoli D, Bernabò N, et al. Retrospective and observational investigation of canine microcytosis in relationship to sex, breed, diseases, and other complete blood count parameters. Comp Clin Path 2010;21(5):545–53.
17. Urrechaga E, Borque L, Escanero JF. Erythrocyte and reticulocyte indices in the assessment of erythropoiesis activity and iron availability. Int J Lab Hematol 2013; 35(2):144–9.
18. Mast AE, Blinder MA, Dietzen DJ. Reticulocyte hemoglobin content. Am J Hematol 2008;83(4):307–10.
19. Fry MM, Kirk CA. Reticulocyte indices in a canine model of nutritional iron deficiency. Vet Clin Pathol 2006;35(2):172–81.
20. Foy DS, Friedrichs KR, Bach JF. Evaluation of Iron Deficiency Using Reticulocyte Indices in Dogs Enrolled in a Blood Donor Program. J Vet Intern Med 2015;29(5): 1376–80.
21. Radakovich LB, Santangelo KS, Olver CS. Reticulocyte hemoglobin content does not differentiate true from functional iron deficiency in dogs. Vet Clin Pathol 2015; 44(4):511–8.
22. Meléndez-Lazo A, Tvarijonaviciute A, Cerón JJ, et al. Evaluation of the relationship between selected reticulocyte parameters and inflammation determined by plasma C-reactive protein in dogs. J Comp Pathol 2015;152(4):304–12.
23. Schaefer DMW, Stokol T. The utility of reticulocyte indices in distinguishing iron deficiency anemia from anemia of inflammatory disease, portosystemic shunting, and breed-associated microcytosis in dogs. Vet Clin Pathol 2015;44(1):109–19.

24. Chikazawa S, Hori Y, Kanai K, et al. Factors influencing measurement of serum iron concentration in dogs: diurnal variation and hyperferritinemia. J Vet Med Sci 2013;75(12):1615–8.
25. Bohn AA. Diagnosis of disorders of iron metabolism in dogs and cats. Vet Clin North Am Small Anim Pract 2013;43(6):1319–30, vii.
26. Stockham SL, Scott MA. Fundamentals of veterinary clinical pathology. 2nd edition. Ames (IA): Blackwell Publishing; 2011.
27. Pietrangelo A. Genetics, genetic testing, and management of hemochromatosis: 15 years since hepcidin. Gastroenterology 2015;149(5):1240–51.e4.
28. Sprague WS, Hackett TB, Johnson JS, et al. Hemochromatosis secondary to repeated blood transfusions in a dog. Vet Pathol 2003;40(3):334–7.
29. Gultekin GI, Raj K, Foureman P, et al. Erythrocytic pyruvate kinase mutations causing hemolytic anemia, osteosclerosis, and seconday hemochromatosis in dogs. J Vet Intern Med 2012;26(4):935–44.
30. Harman D. Lipofuscin and ceroid formation: the cellular recycling system. Adv Exp Med Biol 1989;266:3–15.
31. Riis RC, Cummings JF, Loew ER, et al. Tibetan terrier model of canine ceroid lipofuscinosis. Am J Med Genet 1992;42(4):615–21.

Bone Marrow Aspirate Evaluation

Nicole I. Stacy, DVM, Dr med vet[a],*, John W. Harvey, DVM, PhD[b]

KEYWORDS

• Bone marrow • Cat • Cytology • Dog • Evaluation • Interpretation

KEY POINTS

• Bone marrow aspirate evaluation is a key diagnostic tool in small animal medicine that is used to answer specific questions that cannot be answered by routine diagnostics, such as complete blood cell count (CBC) and serum biochemistry.

• Bone marrow examination typically provides information concerning the likely pathogenesis of cytopenias and other abnormalities in blood.

• Once the pathogenesis of a disorder is determined, a short differential list of specific disorders can be provided, and, in some instances, a specific diagnosis can be made.

• Appropriate sampling and sample preparation techniques are the basis for obtaining high-quality bone marrow specimens. Knowledge of the morphology of bone marrow cells and a systematic approach to the evaluation of bone marrow cytology (in context of a current CBC) are the basis for complete and accurate interpretation of bone marrow cytologic findings.

INTRODUCTION

Bone marrow tissue provides complex microenvironments for the structural and nutritional support essential for orderly differentiation, proliferation, maturation, and release of developing blood cells. The tissue is filled with a network of sinusoids lined by a single layer of endothelial cells. Hematopoietic cells and supporting structures, consisting of adipose tissue, reticular cells, and extracellular matrix, are located outside the vasculature.[1] The bone marrow is structured in distinct and functionally efficient ways. For example, megakaryocytes are located next to sinusoids and extend cytoplasmic processes (proplatelets) into the vasculature, where they bud off to produce platelets. In addition, precursors of the erythroid cell line surround macrophages

The authors have nothing to disclose.
[a] Department of Large Animal Clinical Sciences, College of Veterinary Medicine, University of Florida, 2015 Southwest 16th Avenue, Gainesville, FL 32610, USA; [b] Department of Physiological Sciences, College of Veterinary Medicine, University of Florida, Box 100103, Gainesville, FL 32610, USA
* Corresponding author.
E-mail address: stacyn@ufl.edu

(called erythroid islands) that provide growth factors needed for erythrocyte production. The main function of bone marrow is the production of all blood cell types from primitive stem cells in adult mammals. It responds sensitively to increased peripheral blood cell demands through hematopoietic growth factors and alterations in the bone marrow microenvironment.

Bone marrow aspirate smears provide the best morphologic assessment of hematopoietic cells and determination of cell proportions (**Fig. 1**), that is, the myeloid to erythroid (M:E) ratio and percentages of lymphocytes, plasma cells, macrophages, and mast cells. In contrast, histopathologic evaluation of core biopsies is the best means to evaluate structural and stromal changes and marrow cellularity (**Fig. 2**), for example, diagnosis of myelofibrosis, inflammation, osteolysis, and myelonecrosis, or confirmation of generalized bone marrow hypoplasia or aplasia, which may be difficult diagnoses when the sample quality of a bone marrow aspirate is questionable. Bone marrow aspirate biopsies are more frequently performed than core biopsies in small animal practice because the procedure is faster, easier to perform, and less expensive. Both complement each other, however, in complete evaluation of the bone marrow and the diagnosis of its disorders.

The goal of this article is to provide an overview of bone marrow aspirate evaluation and cytologic interpretation. Readers are referred to recommended references for additional reading.[2–4]

INDICATIONS FOR BONE MARROW ASPIRATION

Bone marrow evaluation is indicated when peripheral blood cell abnormalities are present that cannot be explained in context of clinical history, physical examination, or other additional diagnostics (eg, diagnostic imaging, chemistry). **Box 1** provides an overview of indications for bone marrow aspirate sampling in small animal practice, based on Harvey[2] and Raskin.[3]

Contraindications for bone marrow aspirate and core biopsy sampling should be considered before performing these procedures on a patient. The main consideration is whether an aspirate and/or core biopsy is truly indicated. Procedural risks, including restraint, sedation, and anesthesia (when used), are generally minimal, unless a patient

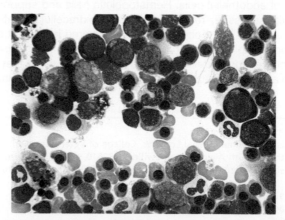

Fig. 1. Bone marrow aspirate from a dog with erythroid hyperplasia demonstrating the morphologic detail of hematopoietic cells, which can be visualized by cytologic evaluation (Wright-Giemsa stain, original magnification ×50).

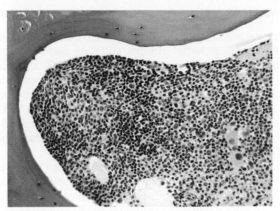

Fig. 2. Bone marrow core biopsy from a dog exhibiting an infiltrate of small lymphocytes consistent with CLL (hematoxylin-eosin stain, original magnification ×10).

is severely ill. Postprocedural hemorrhage in patients with bleeding disorders and in patients with monoclonal hyperglobulinemias is rare and not life-threatening. In addition, postprocedural infection is rare, even in neutropenic patients, if proper aseptic technique is used.[2]

Box 1
Indications for bone marrow aspirate collection in dogs and cats

Persistent neutropenia without evidence of regeneration[a]

Unexplained thrombocytopenia[a]

Nonregenerative or poorly regenerative anemia[a]

Bicytopenia/pancytopenia

Persistent thrombocytosis

Persistent leukocytosis (especially lymphocytosis with circulating atypical lymphocytes)

Abnormal blood cell morphology or abnormal cells in circulation (suspicion of hematopoietic neoplasia)

Unexplained presence of immature cells in blood (eg, leukoerythroblastosis)

Staging of lymphoma or mast cell tumors[a]

Assessment of body iron stores in dogs

Suspicion of osteomyelitis or infiltrative bone marrow disease

Unexplained hypercalcemia (potentially associated with lymphoid neoplasia, multiple myeloma, or metastatic neoplasia to bone)

Unexplained hyperproteinemia (if suspicion of multiple myeloma, lymphoma, leishmaniasis, or fungal infection)

Monoclonal (or rarely biclonal) hyperglobulinemia (eg, plasma cell neoplasia or B-cell CLL)

Diagnostic work-up in patients with fever of unknown origin, unexplained weight loss, or unexplained malaise

  [a] Frequent indications.

BONE MARROW ASPIRATION AND BONE MARROW SMEAR PREPARATION

Preferred bone marrow aspiration sites include the proximal end of the humerus (in animals older than 6 months) or femur in dogs and cats and the iliac crest, mainly in dogs.[2,3] The sternum may be suitable in dogs the size of Beagles or larger, using a 1-inch 20-gauge or 22-gauge hypodermic needle.[5] All listed sites except for the proximal femur are also suitable for bone marrow core biopsy.[2] A 16-gauge or 18-gauge Rosenthal or Illinois bone marrow aspiration needle with 1-inch to 1.5-inch length is recommended for bone marrow aspiration, whereas a larger Jamshidi needle provides good results with bone marrow core biopsies. Details on the procedure of bone marrow sampling are provided by Harvey[2] and Raskin.[3]

A bone marrow aspirate is only diagnostically useful when the sample is representative of the tissue/lesion and a high-quality smear preparation is made. Because bone marrow samples tend to clot rapidly and cells degenerate quickly, slides need to be prepared immediately after sample collection, or the bone marrow may be collected directly into a syringe with several drops of 4% of the anticoagulant ethylenediaminetetraacetic acid (EDTA).[2] EDTA preservation allows for additional time during sample collection to obtain a sufficient specimen, but slides should also be prepared quickly after sample collection to avoid cell degeneration.[2] Immediately after well mixing of bone marrow with anticoagulant in the syringe, the sample is expelled onto a slide or Petri dish where bone marrow particles become visible as small white flecks. These flecks tend to stick to the bottom of the Petri dish and can be separated from contaminating blood by tilting the Petri dish and collecting the flecks with a capillary tube or pipette for slide preparation. If the flecks are expelled onto a slide, they tend to stick to the spot of initial contact with the slide, and they can be separated from blood by holding the slide vertically, which allows blood to run off. Then a second glass slide or coverslip slide can be placed across the sample slide and carefully smeared using a squash technique.[2] It is recommended to prepare multiple slides (eg, minimum of 5 slides). Slides should be rapidly and completely air dried and can then be stained with Romanowsky-type stains, including Wright, Giemsa, Wright-Giemsa, and Diff-Quik. Staining times are generally longer for bone marrow cytology smears compared with blood films because they are much thicker. After staining, bone marrow flecks become visible as blue-staining areas on the slide. For assessment of bone marrow iron stores, staining of 1 slide with the Prussian blue reaction is helpful in dogs (**Fig. 3**). Some slides may be kept aside unstained for special stains or other additional diagnostics (discussed later).

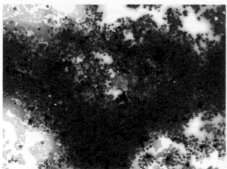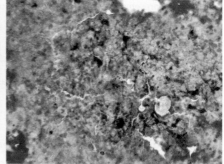

Fig. 3. Bone marrow aspirate of a dog with anemia of inflammatory disease exhibiting abundant black globular material with Wright-Giemsa stain (original magnification ×10) consistent with hemosiderin (*left*) and abundant corresponding blue-staining material with Prussian blue reaction (*right*).

In addition to bone marrow aspirate smears, a core biopsy may be carefully rolled onto a glass slide with a second slide if a nondiagnostic or poorly cellular bone marrow aspirate is obtained. The core biopsy is then placed in 10% buffered formalin. The formalin-containing sample container needs to be packed tightly and away from bone marrow and blood films during shipment, because formalin fumes may damage them.

SYSTEMATIC APPROACH TO CYTOLOGIC EVALUATION OF BONE MARROW ASPIRATES

A systematic approach to bone marrow aspirate evaluation is the basis for a complete and accurate interpretation of qualitative and semiquantitative bone marrow cytologic findings. Proper cell identification is crucial for cytologic evaluation.

Morphology of the Erythroid Cell Line

Compared with the granulocytic cell line, erythroid precursors are generally smaller, exhibit more distinctly spherical nuclei with more condensed dark nuclear chromatin, and have darker cytoplasm that can be deeply basophilic in the early-stage precursors (rubriblasts, prorubricytes, and basophilic rubricytes) (**Fig. 4**). As erythroid precursors mature, they become smaller, the nuclei progressively condense, and the cytoplasm changes from basophilic to pink/orange due to accumulation of synthesized hemoglobin. When cell maturation is orderly, the nucleus is extruded before cells fully mature, resulting in the formation of a reticulocyte.[2] Immature erythroid cell stages include rubriblasts and prorubricytes and should be less than or equal to 5% of all nucleated cells, whereas basophilic rubricytes, polychromatophilic rubricytes, and metarubricytes are considered mature nucleated erythroid stages. The presence or absence of polychromatophilic erythrocytes (reticulocytes) is noted, but these cells are not counted in the M:E ratio.

Morphology of the Granulocytic Cell Line

Compared with erythroid precursors, the larger paler cells with finer chromatin and gray cytoplasm generally represent granulocytic precursors. As granulocytic precursors mature, they reduce somewhat in size, the nucleus condenses and undergoes shape changes, the cytoplasmic color changes from pale grey-basophilic to nearly colorless in neutrophils, primary cytoplasmic granules become invisible in promyelocytes, and secondary cytoplasmic granules become evident starting at the myelocyte stage as colorless (neutrophils), red (eosinophils), or blue (basophils) (see **Fig. 4**; **Fig. 5**). Immature myeloid cell stages, including myeloblasts and promyelocytes, should comprise less than or equal to 5% of all nucleated cells, whereas mature myeloid stages are represented by myelocytes, metamyelocytes, band cells, and mature neutrophils, eosinophils, and basophils.

Morphology of the Megakaryocytic Cell Line

Megakaryoblasts may be difficult to differentiate from precursors of other cell lines, whereas the following maturation stages are easier to identify: promegakaryocytes with 2 to 4 nuclei produced through endomitosis and deeply basophilic cytoplasm, basophilic megakaryocytes with multiple fused nuclei and basophilic cytoplasm, and the larger mature megakaryocytes with multiple fused nuclei and abundant cytoplasm filled with magenta-colored granules (**Fig. 6**).[1,2] The megakaryocytic cell line is the only hemic cell line that undergoes endomitosis and enlarges during maturation.[1]

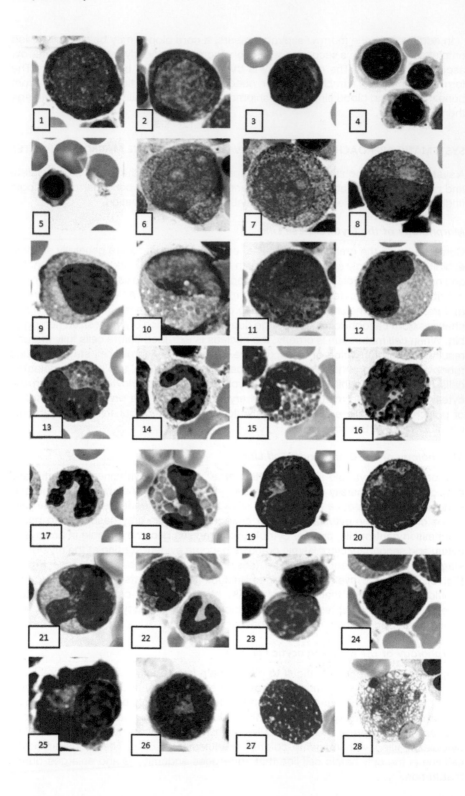

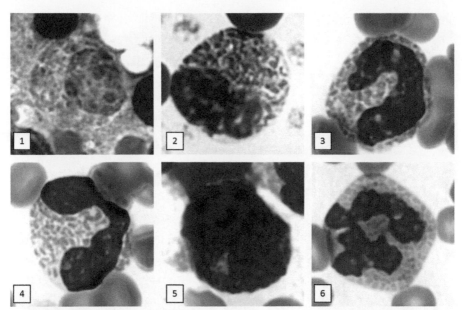

Fig. 5. Bone marrow aspirates and blood films of cats with stages of eosinophil and basophil maturation (Wright-Giemsa stain, original magnification ×100). 1, eosinophilic myelocyte. 2, eosinophilic metamyelocyte. 3, band eosinophil. 4, segmented (mature) eosinophil. 5, basophilic myelocyte. 6, segmented (mature) basophil. Images of metamyelocyte and band basophil are not shown.

Fig. 4. Image composite of hemic cells in canine bone marrow stained with Wright-Giemsa stain (original magnification ×100). 1, Rubriblast with diffusely coarse chromatin, nucleoli, and deeply basophilic cytoplasm. 2, Prorubricyte with diffusely coarse chromatin, absence of nucleoli, and basophilic cytoplasm. 3, Basophilic rubricyte with clumped chromatin and blue cytoplasm. 4, Polychromatophilic rubricytes with dense clumped chromatin and polychromatophilic cytoplasm. 5, Metarubricyte (nucleated), reticulocyte (*right*) after extrusion of the nucleus, and mature erythrocyte (*top of image*). 6, Myeloblast with reticular chromatin, prominent nucleoli, and blue cytoplasm. 7, Type III myeloblast with prominent nucleoli and blue cytoplasm with frequent pink staining granules 8, Promyelocyte with reticular chromatin and blue cytoplasm with frequent pink staining granules. 9, Neutrophilic myelocyte with clumped chromatin and light blue cytoplasm. 10, Eosinophilic myelocyte with finely clumped chromatin and pale to medium basophilic cytoplasm filled with eosinophilic granules. 11, Basophilic myelocyte with finely clumped chromatin and medium basophilic cytoplasm filled with purple granules. 12, Neutrophilic metamyelocyte with kidney-shaped nucleus and lightly basophilic cytoplasm. 13, Eosinophilic metamyelocyte with kidney-shaped nucleus and medium basophilic cytoplasm filled with eosinophilic granules. 14, Band neutrophil. 15, Band eosinophil. 16, Band basophil. 17, Mature segmented neutrophil. 18, Mature segmented eosinophil. 19, Monoblast with kidney-shaped nucleus containing nucleoli and deeply basophilic cytoplasm. 20, Presumed promonocyte with deeply basophilic cytoplasm. 21, Mature monocyte. 22, Mature monocyte (*left*) and band neutrophil (*right*). 23, Small lymphocyte and polychromatophilic rubricyte. 24, Presumptive prolymphocyte. 25, Plasma cell. 26, Mitotic figure in polychromatophilic rubricyte. 27, Free nucleus of a lysed cells with visible nucleoli. 28, Reddish staining material consistent with free nucleus of a lysed cell (so-called basket cell although no cytoplasm present).

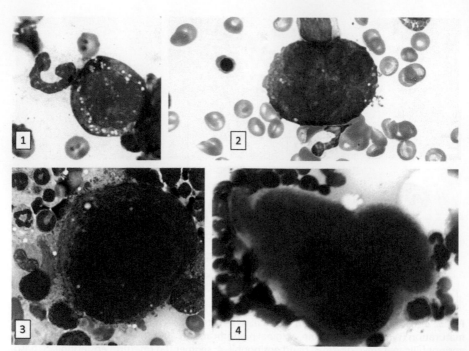

Fig. 6. Megakaryocyte cell line in bone marrow aspirate smears of dogs (Wright-Giemsa stain, original magnification ×50). 1, Megakaryoblast with 1 nucleus. 2, Promegakaryocyte with multiple nuclei. 3, Basophilic megakaryocyte with fused nuclei. 4, Mature megakaryocyte with granular cytoplasm.

Morphology of the Monocytic Cell Line

The monocytic cell line accounts for a low percentage of cells (≤2% of all nucleated cells). Although the early stages (monoblasts and promonocytes) are difficult to differentiate from other granulocytic precursors, mature monocytes are identical to those observed in the peripheral blood (see **Fig. 4**). Macrophages in the bone marrow may contain phagocytized nucleoproteinaceous debris, hemosiderin, and rarely erythrocytes or leukocytes in normal animals. Although macrophages frequently are located within the center of erythroid islands surrounded by erythroid precursors, erythroid islands may not necessarily be evident in bone marrow aspirates due to disruption during bone marrow aspiration and smear preparation.

Morphology of Lymphocytes and Plasma Cells

Because bone marrow is a lymphoid organ and lymphocytes also develop in this complex tissue, low numbers of lymphoblasts and prolymphocytes and variable numbers of mature lymphocytes are present in normal bone marrow (see **Fig. 4**). Plasma cells are typical in appearance as observed in other lymphoid tissues (see **Fig. 4**). They have a single often eccentrically positioned spherical nucleus, a perinuclear Golgi zone, and deeply basophilic cytoplasm. They may exhibit a reddish periphery (so-called flame cells). Plasma cells may be increased with antigenic stimulation (normal morphology) or in multiple myeloma with nuclear features of malignancy (**Fig. 7**). They may contain pale basophilic or pink inclusions that are round, needle-like, or coalescing (so-called Mott cells) as observed with conditions of antigenic stimulation.

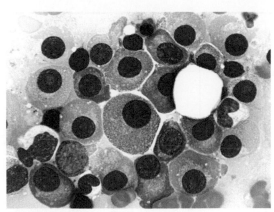

Fig. 7. Bone marrow aspirate of a dog with neoplastic plasma cells exhibiting anisokaryosis, anisocytosis, and prominent nucleoli, consistent with multiple myeloma (Wright-Giemsa stain, original magnification ×50).

Osteoclasts and Osteoblasts

Osteoclasts are large multinucleated cells with individual nuclei (in contrast to fused nuclei in megakaryocytes), magenta cytoplasmic granules, and cytoplasmic trails, whereas osteoblasts are oval with a single, often oval eccentric nucleus with finely stippled chromatin, pale to medium basophilic, sometimes foamy cytoplasm, and Golgi zone that may be perinuclear. The significance of their presence in bone marrow aspirates is indicated in **Table 1**.

Miscellaneous Cells and Mitotic Figures

Free nuclei of lysed cells are always observed in bone marrow aspirate smears (see **Fig. 4**). Adipocytes appear as large empty vacuoles after alcohol fixation. Stromal cells and capillaries are sometimes seen. Mast cells are rarely seen in normal bone marrow. They have a round nucleus and are filled with numerous small round purple granules.

Because cells continuously develop in the bone marrow throughout adult life, bone marrow tissue can contain several mitotic figures; up to 2% of nucleated cells (see **Fig. 4**).[2]

Systematic Approach to the Cytologic Evaluation of Bone Marrow Aspirates

An overview of consecutive steps for the systematic evaluation of bone marrow aspirates based on Harvey[2] is presented in **Table 1**.

INTERPRETATION OF BONE MARROW FINDINGS

Bone marrow aspirate findings are interpreted in context of history, clinical findings, hematology and chemistry data, and additional diagnostic tests. Current CBC results (at time or within 24 hours of bone marrow collection), including a blood film, are essential for the proper interpretation of the M:E ratio in context of bone marrow cellularity.[3] The M:E ratio ranges from 0.75 to 2.53 (mean 1.25) in dogs and from 1.21 to 2.16 (mean 1.63) in cats.[6] For example, an increased M:E ratio may indicate myeloid hyperplasia, erythroid hypoplasia, or a combination of both. Possible cytologic interpretations of M:E ratios are given in **Box 2**, which shows that information from the CBC (especially the neutrophil count and degree of left shift [when present]) and hematocrit with reticulocyte count (if anemic) and/or valid information concerning the overall

Table 1
An overview of a systematic approach to bone marrow aspirate evaluation based on Harvey[2]

Step	Goal/Comments
Scanning with low-power objectives	Normal: heterogenous appearance (blood cell precursors, blood vessels, reticular cells, macrophages, plasma cells) • Homogenous appearance: likely abnormal population of cells Impression on overall cellularity Impression on megakaryocyte number Fat: dissolved during alcohol fixation and visible as variably sized clear areas
Evaluation of bone marrow cellularity	Evaluate overall cellularity of specimen, cell distributions, and cellularity of bone marrow particles Evaluate as many particles as possible • Estimation of proportions of hematopoietic cells and fat within marrow particles • Normal: 1/3–2/3 cells (depending on age of animal: cellularity decreases with age) >75% Cells: hypercellular >75% Fat: hypocellular If insufficient particles on aspirate smear, it is impossible to accurately estimate marrow cellularity Increased cellularity → increased proliferation of one or more cell types • Increased peripheral need, anemia, inflammation • Secondary to dysplastic or neoplastic proliferations or infiltration of neoplastic cells from peripheral tissues (eg, metastasis)
Megakaryocytes	Evaluation of frequency: evaluate 20–25 × 10 objective fields Each bone marrow particle should have several associated megakaryocytes • 5–15 Per particle likely normal • >15 Likely increased • <5 Likely decreased Evaluation of maturation • Orderly and synchronous? (>80%–90% should be mature) • Complete? Evaluation of morphology • Normal? • Abnormal morphology? (eg, dwarf megakaryocytes)

Erythroid cell line	Evaluate maturation • Orderly and synchronous? • Complete? • Adequate degree of polychromatophilic erythrocytes present? Evaluate morphology • Normal? • Abnormal? (eg, megaloblastic cells, binucleated cells, or pleomorphic nuclei) Rubriblasts and prorubricytes should be ≤5% of all nucleated cells Increased: suggestive of hyperplasia, neoplasia, or maturation abnormality
Granulocytic cells	Evaluate maturation • Orderly and synchronous? • Complete? Evaluate morphology • Normal? • Abnormal? (eg, nuclear dysplasia) Myeloblasts and promyelocytes should be ≤5% of all nucleated cells Increased: suggestive of hyperplasia, neoplasia, or maturation abnormality Eosinophils <6%; basophils ≤1% Increases • Inflammation • Myeloid neoplasms
M:E	Definition: ratio of granulocytic cells (including mature cells) to nucleated erythroid cells 500 Differential cell count (count cells in close proximity to particles and on different smears [eg, 100 cells per smear]) CBC results of concurrent blood sample essential for interpretation Dilution of peripheral blood can have an effect, especially with neutrophilia Normal in dogs: 0.75–2.5; cats 1–3
Lymphocytes	Generally <10% Can be up to 14% in healthy dogs, up to 20% in healthy cats Evaluate morphology Increased • CLL (often diffuse distribution) • Erythroid aplasia • Immune-mediated nonregenerative anemia, pure red cell aplasia • Antigenic stimulation (eg, ehrlichiosis [dogs]) griseofulvin toxicosis, systemic lupus erythematosus) • Cats: thymoma, cholangiohepatitis • Increased immature lymphocytes: acute lymphoblastic leukemia or metastatic lymphoma

(continued on next page)

Table 1
(continued)

Step	Goal/Comments
Plasma cells	Normal: ≤2%; often associated with bone marrow particles Increased: ≥3% • Multiple myeloma • Immune-mediated hemolytic anemia • Erythroid aplasia • Dogs: *Ehrlichia canis* infection, leishmaniasis, myelodysplasia, estrogen-induced bone marrow damage, rarely with myelodysplasia • Cats: feline infectious peritonitis
Mononuclear phagocytes	Normal: ≤2% (generally not >1%) Increased • Inflammation/infection, necrosis • Myeloid neoplasia (typically with high increases) • Histiocytic sarcoma Phagocytosis of erythroid stages • Primary or secondary immune-mediated anemia • Hemoparasites (eg, *Babesia, Cytauxzoon, Leishmania, Trypanosoma,* and Hemoplasma spp) • Hemophagocytic histiocytic sarcoma • Hemophagocytic syndrome • After blood transfusion • Acquired and congenital dyserythropoiesis Leukophagocytosis (rare) • Immune-mediated neutropenia • Myeloid neoplasms • Hemophagocytic syndrome Phagocytosis of cellular debris • Bone marrow necrosis

Other cell types and findings	Mitotic figures • Should be ≤2% of nucleated cells • In erythroid and myeloid hyperplasia, acute leukemias • Dramatic increase: as soon as hours after vincristine administration • Congenital dyserythropoiesis Osteoclasts, osteoblasts • Often present in young growing animals, rare in adults • Increased in adults with bone remodeling (eg, increased parathyroid hormone, osteosarcoma) Mast cells • Rare in normal bone marrow • Increased: aplastic anemia of various etiologies, inflammation, metastatic mast cells tumors, cat: noncutaneous systemic mastocytosis Increased reticular stromal cells ± collagen • Stromal hyperplasia and/or myelofibrosis (core biopsy recommended for confirmation) Metastatic cells • From nonhematopoietic sarcomas or carcinomas Screen carefully for infectious agents (eg, bacteria, protozoa, and fungi)
Stainable iron (Prussian blue reaction)	Evaluate at least 9 particles for adequate assessment of marrow hemosiderin stores in bone marrow macrophages: blue-grey to black granular material (Wright-Giemsa stain) or blue to blue-green (Prussian blue stain) often in macrophages or extracellularly Cats: lack stainable iron (cannot be used for diagnosis of iron deficiency anemia) • Presence is abnormal, possible with myeloid dysplasia or neoplasia, hemolytic anemia, after blood transfusion Dogs • Low iron stores in weaned dogs at the end of nursing period • Increase with age Increased with • Hemolytic anemia • Dyserythropoiesis (often concurrent erythrophagocytosis) • Decreased blood cell production (including anemia of inflammatory or chronic disease, persistent nonregenerative anemia) • Repeated blood transfusions Decreased with • Iron deficiency anemia (dog) • Possibly absent with polycythemia vera (dog)

Adapted from Harvey JW. Veterinary hematology: a diagnostic guide and color atlas. St Louis (MO): Elsevier Saunders; 2012; with permission.

Box 2
Possible cytologic interpretations of myeloid to erythroid ratios

Normal myeloid to erythroid ratio

Normal myeloid and erythroid production

Both myeloid and erythroid hyperplasia
   Bone marrow cellularity increased
   Possible CBC findings
      Neutrophilia (effective granulopoiesis)
      Neutropenia (ineffective granulopoiesis)
      Regenerative anemia (effective erythropoiesis; (eg, iron-deficiency anemia, immune-mediated hemolytic anemia)
      Nonregenerative anemia (ineffective erythropoiesis)

Both myeloid and erythroid hypoplasia
   Bone marrow cellularity decreased
   Possible CBC findings
      Nonregenerative anemia
      Neutropenia
      Thrombocytopenia
      Pancytopenia

High myeloid to erythroid ratio

Myeloid hyperplasia
   Bone marrow cellularity normal or increased
   Possible CBC findings
      Neutrophilia with left-shift (effective granulopoiesis)
      Neutropenia (ineffective granulopoiesis)
      Nonregenerative anemia
      Thrombocytosis secondary to chronic inflammation
      If abnormal cells in circulation: consider acute or CML

Erythroid hypoplasia
   Bone marrow cellularity normal or decreased
   Possible CBC findings
      Nonregenerative anemia

Combination of the above

Low myeloid to erythroid ratio

Erythroid hyperplasia
   Bone marrow cellularity normal or increased
   Possible CBC findings
      Regenerative anemia (effective erythropoiesis)
      Nonregenerative anemia (ineffective erythropoiesis)
      Leukocyte counts variable
      If abnormal erythroid cells in circulation: consider MDS-erythroid (<20% blasts), erythroleukemia (≥20% blasts)

Myeloid hypoplasia
   Bone marrow cellularity normal or decreased
   Possible CBC findings
      Neutropenia

Combination of the above

---

marrow cellularity is/are needed to differentiate the possibilities. The morphology and distribution of the maturational stages in leukocyte and erythroid cell lines along with CBC data allow for subdivisions to be made within these interpretations. Because a detailed discussion of bone marrow findings and their interpretation is beyond this publication, the following serves as an overview of commonly encountered disorders and conditions in small animal practice.

Hypocellular Bone Marrow and Hypoplasia of Hemic Cell Lines

If a bone marrow aspirate is hypocellular, considerations include the presence of a nonrepresentative specimen (ie, bone marrow spicules absent), aplastic bone marrow/generalized marrow hypoplasia, myelofibrosis, and myelonecrosis. A reaspiration attempt and/or core bone marrow biopsy may be necessary to confirm generalized marrow hypoplasia, which is often accompanied by peripheral pancytopenia. Generalized bone marrow hypoplasia or aplasia is present when all cell lines are markedly reduced or absent. Several causes have been associated with this condition, including infections (eg, ehrlichiosis and parvovirus), various drugs, toxins, and neoplasia.[2] Estrogen-secreting tumors or estrogen administration can cause aplastic anemia in dogs, but it has not been reported in cats. With myelofibrosis, a dry tap or a specimen with low cellularity and well-differentiated mesenchymal cells may be obtained.[2] Myelonecrosis is characterized by the presence of lysed nucleoproteinaceous material that may be phagocytized by macrophages and is caused by bone marrow damage through ischemia or various causes of direct damage to developing precursor cells.[2]

Selective erythroid or granulocytic hypoplasia is caused by decreased cell production of the respective cell line. In many disorders or conditions with selective hypoplasia, the precursor cells may be normal or increased, but cells may not mature properly or die before complete maturation within the bone marrow, which is termed *ineffective hematopoiesis*. This diagnosis can only be made by evaluation of the current CBC of a patient, for example, myeloid hyperplasia with severe neutropenia, as can be seen with immune-mediated neutropenia (ineffective granulopoiesis), whereas myeloid hyperplasia with neutrophilia is consistent with inflammation and effective granulopoiesis (**Fig. 8**). Ineffective hematopoiesis may be transient in many conditions (eg, bone marrow injury) and a bone marrow aspirate may reflect a preregenerative or early regenerative response.

Selective erythroid hypoplasia (**Fig. 9**) or granulocytic hypoplasia (**Fig. 10**) has been observed with immune-mediated precursor destruction, drug toxicities, and infections (eg, granulocytic hypoplasia with parvovirus infection in dogs and cats, erythroid

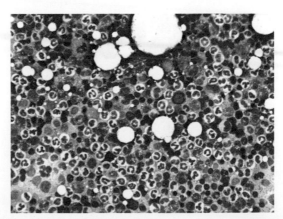

Fig. 8. Neutrophilic and eosinophilic hyperplasia in a bone marrow aspirate of a dog (Wright-Giemsa stain, original magnification ×20).

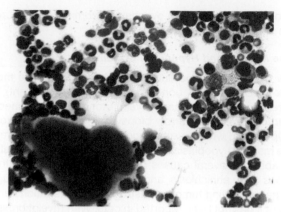

Fig. 9. Bone marrow aspirate from a dog with red cell aplasia (Wright-Giemsa stain, original magnification ×20).

hypoplasia in cats with feline leukemia virus [FeLV] infection). Additional causes for selective erythroid hypoplasia include anemia of inflammation, endocrine disorders, and renal disease.[2] Selective megakaryocytic hypoplasia may be associated with immune-mediated destruction or effects from various drugs and toxins.[2]

Hypercellular Bone Marrow and Hyperplasia of Hemic Cell Lines

Hyperplasia results from an increased number of cells of one or more cell lines in the bone marrow as a result of a response to peripheral demand, dysplasia, or neoplasia. Commonly observed conditions in small animal practice associated with erythroid hyperplasia and regenerative anemia (**Fig. 11**) include hemorrhagic or hemolytic anemia, cardiac or pulmonary disease, or inappropriate erythropoietin production as result of various renal disease.[2] Ineffective erythroid hyperplasia, characterized by nonregenerative anemia, may be associated with immune-mediated disease (eg, observation of phagocytosis of erythroid precursors by bone marrow macrophages), various nutritional deficiencies, or myelodysplastic syndrome (MDS)-erythroid. Inflammation, infection, necrosis, and early-stage estrogen-induced bone marrow toxicosis may

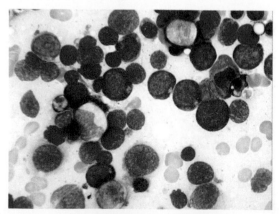

Fig. 10. Bone marrow aspirate of a dog with transient granulocytic hypoplasia (Wright-Giemsa stain, original magnification ×50).

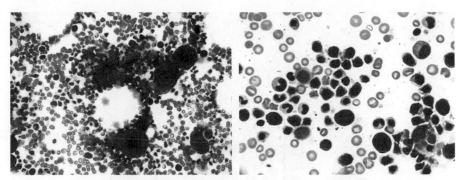

Fig. 11. Bone marrow aspirate of a dog with regenerative immune-mediated hemolytic anemia with erythroid and megakaryocytic hyperplasia and erythrophagia after a recent blood transfusion (*bottom right corner of both images*) (Wright-Giemsa stain, original magnification ×10 [*left*], ×20 [*right*]).

result in effective myeloid hyperplasia (see **Fig. 8**) with peripheral neutrophilia, whereas ineffective granulopoiesis is characterized by myeloid hyperplasia and neutropenia (**Figs. 12** and **13**), as can be seen with septicemic marrow injury, immune-mediated conditions, various drug toxicities, MDSs, and sometimes acute myelogenous leukemia (AML). MDS is most common in cats with FeLV or feline immunodeficiency virus infections.[2]

Megakaryocytic hyperplasia (**Fig. 14**) is the result of stimulation of megakaryopoiesis and is frequently observed with recovery from various conditions that previously resulted in thrombocytopenia (eg, disseminated intravascular coagulation [DIC] or immune-mediated thrombocytopenia), inflammation, iron-deficiency anemia, or essential thrombocythemia. Thrombocytopenia with megakaryocytic hyperplasia can be seen with immune-mediated platelet destruction, increased peripheral utilization (DIC, endothelial injury, and infections), and hypersplenism.

Myelodysplasia

Myelodysplasia is characterized by dysplastic nuclear changes in 1 or more cell lines in bone marrow and a possible increase of blast cells (less than 20% of nucleated

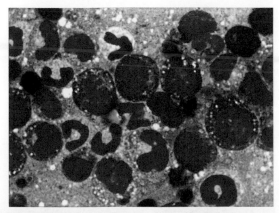

Fig. 12. Myeloid hyperplasia with a toxic left shift in a bone marrow aspirate from a dog with a severe toxic neutropenia in blood that appeared to be secondary to septicemia (Wright-Giemsa stain, original magnification ×100).

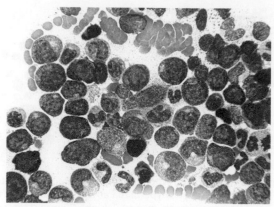

Fig. 13. Bone marrow aspirate of a cat with myeloid hyperplasia and left shift in an early response to a peripheral neutropenia (Wright-Giemsa stain, original magnification ×50).

cells). Bone marrow and CBC findings supporting the interpretation of myelodysplasia can be variable and may present with peripheral cytopenias, overt dysplastic changes in blood and in bone marrow cell lines, and normal or increased bone marrow cellularity with ineffective hematopoiesis.[2,7] Possible cytologic abnormalities characterizing dysplastic changes include megaloblastic erythroid cells (**Fig. 15**), giant neutrophilic cells, abnormally segmented or hyposegmented neutrophils (**Fig. 16**), and/or dwarf megakaryocytes (**Fig. 17**).[2] MDSs result from acquired genetic defects and are further classified into subtypes based on blast percentages and M:E ratio; they may progress to acute leukemias (eg, AML in dogs and cats) or lymphoid neoplasms in FeLV-infected cats.[2] MDSs need to be differentiated from secondary myelodysplasia, which is typically associated with certain diseases or toxins.[2,7]

Neoplasia

Hemic cell neoplasia is classified into myeloid and lymphoid neoplasias, which are further differentiated into acute and chronic subtypes.[2] Nonhematopoietic neoplasms,

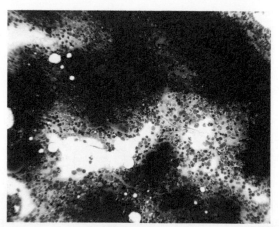

Fig. 14. Bone marrow aspirate of a dog with generalized hyperplasia and prominent megakaryocytic hyperplasia (Wright-Giemsa stain, original magnification ×10).

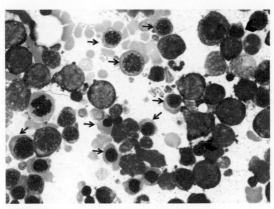

Fig. 15. Bone marrow aspirate of a cat with AML-M6Er (erythroleukemia): megaloblastic precursors (*arrows*) and erythroid precursors with bilobulated nucleus (*arrowheads*) (Wright-Giemsa stain, original magnification ×50).

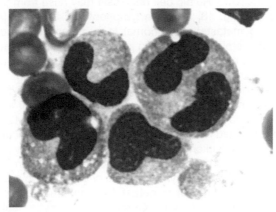

Fig. 16. Bone marrow aspirate of a dog with dysgranulopoeisis as characterized by giant neutrophil precursors with abnormal nuclear morphology (Wright-Giemsa stain, original magnification ×100).

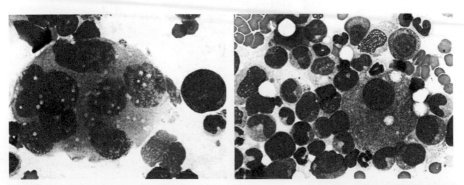

Fig. 17. Dwarf megakaryocytes in the bone marrow of a dog (*left*), and a cat (*right*) with myelodysplasia (Wright-Giemsa stain, original magnification ×50).

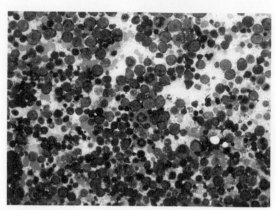

Fig. 18. Bone marrow aspirate of a cat with AML-M6Er (erythroleukemia) (Wright-Giemsa stain, original magnification ×20).

such as various carcinomas, melanoma, mesothelioma, and nephroblastoma, may spread to the bone marrow.[2] Hemic cell neoplasia may arise from the bone marrow (eg, AML [see **Fig. 15; Fig. 18**] or acute lymphoblastic leukemia [ALL]) or spread to the bone marrow (eg, metastatic lymphoma). In the presence of frequent blast cells, the diagnosis of acute hemic cell neoplasia is easily achieved; however, determining the cell of origin may be challenging and additional diagnostics are often needed for further diagnostic information (discussed later).

If the blast percentage of nonlymphoid hemic cells in blood or bone marrow exceeds 20%, a diagnosis of AML is made.[2,7] AML can be further subdivided based on the type(s) of blast cells present. Chronic myeloid leukemia (CML) is characterized by the presence of a marked left shift in blood, which can be difficult to differentiate from inflammation-induced leukemoid reactions. The bone marrow in CML is characterized by granulocytic hyperplasia with a left shift but with less than 20% myeloblasts.

The presence of large numbers of lymphoblasts or prolymphocytes in bone marrow is consistent with either ALL (**Fig. 19**) or metastatic lymphoma. A lack of peripheral tumors supports a diagnosis of ALL. Chronic lymphocytic leukemia (CLL) is

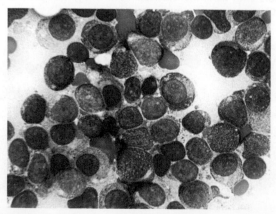

Fig. 19. Acute lymphoblastic leukemia in a bone marrow aspirate of a dog (Wright-Giemsa stain, original magnification ×50).

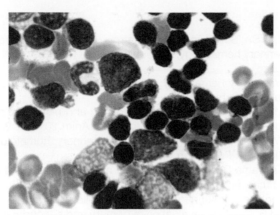

Fig. 20. Bone marrow aspirate from a dog with CLL containing 78% small lymphocytes. The blood lymphocyte count was 78,440/μL (Wright-Giemsa stain, original magnification ×50).

characterized by high mature lymphocyte numbers in blood (**Fig. 20**). The bone marrow usually contains increased numbers of mature lymphocytes; however, T-lymphocyte CLL develops outside the bone marrow (often in the spleen) and may not have infiltrated the marrow when sampled early in disease.

Additional Diagnostics

Saving few unstained slides until completion of cytologic bone marrow evaluation by regular stains can be helpful in cases of need for additional stains to obtain further diagnostic information. Cytochemical staining for the differentiation of myeloid neoplasms and immunocytochemical staining for determination of the lymphoid cell of origin can be useful directly on bone marrow aspirate smears.[8–10] Immunophenotyping of blood and/or bone marrow using flow cytometry with validated antibodies is, however, currently the most frequently used diagnostic tool to diagnose lymphoid and myeloid leukemias.[10,11] Clonality assays using polymerase chain reaction (PCR) have been developed to differentiate reactive from neoplastic lymphoid cell proliferations.[10] PCR can also be useful to identify genetic abnormalities (eg, myeloid leukemia) or infectious agents (eg, rickettsial), whereas histochemical stains can be helpful for diagnosis or confirmation of infectious agents, for example, acid fast-stain for *Mycobacterium* spp and related organisms, and Gomori methenamine silver stain for yeast or fungal organisms. Another histochemical stain used infrequently on bone marrow aspirates is alcian blue at pH 2.5. Positive staining supports the presence of acid mucopolysaccharides and the diagnosis of gelatinous transformation of bone marrow.[2]

SUMMARY

Obtaining and processing a high-quality bone marrow aspirate from a patient with a suspected hematologic disorder provides the basis for accurate cytologic bone marrow aspirate evaluation. Submission of the bone marrow specimen, along with current CBC and chemistry results, a blood film from the current CBC, and a thorough history to a board-certified clinical pathologist for final review can confirm or modify the findings from initial review. Additionally, review by a clinical pathologist may provide additional interpretative information and guidance for further diagnostic testing.

REFERENCES

1. Sharkey LC, Hill SA. Structure of bone marrow. In: Weiss DJ, Wardrop KJ, editors. Schalm's veterinary hematology. 6th edition. Ames (IA): Blackwell Publishing Ltd; 2010. p. 8–13.
2. Harvey JW. Veterinary hematology: a diagnostic guide and color atlas. St Louis (MO): Elsevier Saunders; 2012.
3. Raskin RE, Messick JB. Bone marrow cytologic and histologic biopsies: indications, technique, and evaluation. Vet Clin Small Anim 2012;42:23–42.
4. Weiss DJ, Wardrop KJ, editors. Schalm's veterinary hematology. 6th edition. Ames (IA): Blackwell Publishing Ltd; 2010.
5. Defarges A, Abrams-Ogg A, Foster RA, et al. Comparison of sternal, iliac, and humeral bone marrow aspiration in Beagle dogs. Vet Clin Pathol 2013;42:170–6.
6. Jain NC. Essentials of veterinary hematology. Philadelphia: Lea & Febiger; 1993.
7. Weiss DJ, Aird B. Cytologic evaluation of primary and secondary myelodysplastic syndromes in the dog. Vet Clin Pathol 2001;30:67–75.
8. Raskin RE. Cytochemical staining. In: Weiss DJ, Wardrop KJ, editors. Schalm's veterinary hematology. 6th edition. Ames (IA): Blackwell Publishing Ltd; 2010. p. 1141–61.
9. Stokol T, Schaefer D, Shuman M, et al. Alkaline phosphatase is a useful cytochemical marker for the diagnosis of acute myelomonocytic and monocytic leukemia in the dog. Vet Clin Pathol 2015;44:79–93.
10. Vernau W, Moore PF. An immunophenotype study of canine leukemias and preliminary assessment of clonality by polymerase chain reaction. Vet Immunol Immunopathol 1999;69:145–64.
11. Villiers EJ, Baines S, Law AM, et al. Identification of acute myeloid leukemia in dogs using flow cytometry with myeloperoxidase, MAC387, and a canine neutrophil-specific antibody. Vet Clin Pathol 2006;35:55–71.

Lymphoid Neoplasia

Correlations Between Morphology and Flow Cytometry

Emily D. Rout, DVM[a], Paul R. Avery, VMD, PhD[b],*

KEYWORDS

• Canine • Cytology • Flow cytometry • Immunophenotype • Leukemia • Lymphoma

KEY POINTS

- Major types of canine leukemia and lymphoma include B-cell chronic lymphocytic leukemia, CD8 T-cell chronic lymphocytic leukemia, acute leukemia, diffuse large B-cell lymphoma, CD4 T-cell lymphoma, and T-zone lymphoma/leukemia.
- These major types of canine leukemia and lymphoma often have some characteristic cytologic features, which may aid in directing the subsequent diagnostic workup.
- Flow cytometry examines cell size, cytoplasmic complexity, and expression of cell surface and intracellular proteins (immunophenotype).
- Flow cytometry is an important tool for diagnosis and further characterization of lymphoma and leukemia.
- Flow cytometric features provide valuable prognostic information for certain types of lymphoma and leukemia.

INTRODUCTION

Cytologic examination is a major component in the diagnosis of lymphoid neoplasia in veterinary medicine. Morphologic features are often enough to assign a general pathologic process, but techniques such as histopathology and flow cytometry can be critical for a more definitive classification. Flow cytometry has become increasingly popular over the past decade for immunophenotyping of lymphoma and leukemia in dogs and cats. Flow cytometric features, such as cell size and expression of specific antigens, can be important prognostic factors for certain types of lymphoproliferative disorders.

Disclosure Statement: The authors have nothing to disclose.
[a] Department of Microbiology, Immunology, and Pathology, College of Veterinary Medicine and Biomedical Sciences, Colorado State University, 314-4 Diagnostic Medicine Center, 200 West Lake Street, 1644 Campus Delivery, Fort Collins, CO 80523-1644, USA; [b] Department of Microbiology, Immunology, and Pathology, College of Veterinary Medicine and Biomedical Sciences, Colorado State University, 309 Diagnostic Medicine Center, 200 West Lake Street, 1644 Campus Delivery, Fort Collins, CO 80523-1644, USA
* Corresponding author.
E-mail address: paul.avery@colostate.edu

Vet Clin Small Anim 47 (2017) 53–70
http://dx.doi.org/10.1016/j.cvsm.2016.07.004
0195-5616/17/© 2016 Elsevier Inc. All rights reserved.

The major types of canine lymphoma and leukemia frequently have characteristic cytomorphology. This review describes these major cytologic findings and the corresponding flow cytometric features important for the diagnosis and prognosis of each of these major types. Significantly less is known about the subtypes of feline lymphoma and leukemia. One study evaluated correlations between lymphoma cytomorphology and prognosis in cats and identified a wide variety of morphology subsets, but flow cytometric features were not evaluated.[1] In an effort to minimize subjective findings, feline lymphoproliferative disease is not covered in this review.

We are not advocating the use of cytomorphology in place of objective immunophenotypic or histologic data; however, there are common forms of canine lymphoproliferative disorders where initial cytologic findings can direct and prioritize subsequent investigations. Additionally, there are known limitations to the isolated use of cytomorphology as well as much that is unknown about the cytomorphology in the less common forms of lymphoma/leukemia.

PRINCIPLES OF FLOW CYTOMETRY
Basic Principles

Flow cytometry characterizes different cell types in a population. It allows for the examination of multiple parameters, including cell surface proteins, intracellular proteins, and the size and complexity of individual cells.

Cells in a single-cell fluid suspension are passed by a laser light source in the flow cytometer. Laser light is scattered by the cells and identified by detectors. A detector in front of the light source measures forward scatter (FS), which is proportional to overall cell size. Detectors to the side measure side scatter (SS), which is proportional to internal cell complexity. FS and SS are useful in separating major cell populations within a peripheral blood sample or lymphoid tissue aspirate (**Fig. 1**). Lymphocyte size determination will be slightly variable across flow cytometers and diagnostic laboratories. FS may be measured on a linear scale or a log scale, causing different size interpretations between institutions.

Cells in a mixed population can also be separated based on the proteins or antigens they express. Proteins on the surface of cells or within the cytoplasm are stained with fluorochrome-labeled antibodies. When the fluorochrome is excited by a laser, light of a certain wavelength is emitted and detected. The amount of light emitted is proportional to the amount of antibody bound, and therefore, the amount of antigen on the cell.

Flow cytometry software allows multiple parameters to be examined at once. For example, a subpopulation may be highlighted and enumerated by drawing a gate around the population of interest. Then, other parameters such as FS and SS can be examined for the particular subpopulation within that gate. Additionally, one subpopulation can be evaluated for expression of multiple surface antigens, as long as the corresponding antibodies are labeled with different fluorochromes.

Lineage Determination

Cell lineage is determined by identification of cell surface antigens. The antibodies commonly used to detect these antigens for routine immunophenotyping of lymphoma and leukemia in the dog are listed in **Table 1**.

Additional antibodies are available for the dog, such as anti-CD61 for megakaryoblasts, but these antibodies are predominantly used for research purposes or specific

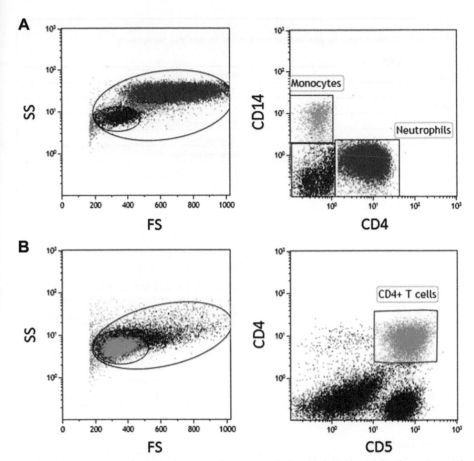

Fig. 1. Flow cytometric features for normal peripheral blood (*A*) and lymph node aspirate (*B*). In the peripheral blood, neutrophils are large with granular cytoplasm, as indicated by high FS and SS (CD4+/CD14−; *magenta*). Monocytes are slightly smaller with less cytoplasmic complexity (CD14+, CD4−; *green*) and small lymphocytes are small with little cytoplasmic complexity (*blue*) and delineated by the small black circle. In a lymph node aspirate, large lymphocytes have forward scatter (FS) and side scatter (SS) properties similar to monocytes. A small black circle is drawn around small lymphocytes (CD4+ lymphocyte subset is *light blue*).

diagnostic cases rather than routine immunophenotyping.[2] A more comprehensive review of the usefulness of flow cytometry for diagnostic and research purposes in veterinary medicine has been discussed elsewhere.[3–5]

For peripheral blood immunophenotyping, the absolute count for each cell subset is determined. For lymph node analysis, the proportion of cells is examined rather than absolute counts. Each diagnostic laboratory must establish their own reference ranges for these values.[6] In normal peripheral blood and lymph node aspirates, there are typically more CD3 T cells than CD21 B cells, and there are typically more CD4 T cells than CD8 T cells.[7–10] The diagnosis of lymphoproliferative disease is then made by establishing that a homogeneous population of cells is expanded beyond the expected reference range, or by identifying a population of cells with an aberrant immunophenotype.[4,5,10–12]

Table 1	
Common antibodies used to phenotype canine hematopoietic neoplasms	
Lymphoid antibodies	
Anti-CD3	T lymphocytes
Anti-CD5	T lymphocytes
Anti-CD4	CD4 T lymphocytes, neutrophils
Anti-CD8	CD8 T lymphocytes
Anti-CD21	B lymphocytes
Anti-CD22	B lymphocytes
Anti-CD79a	B lymphocytes
Anti-Pax5	B lymphocytes
Myeloid antibodies	
Anti-CD14	Monocytes
Anti-CD18	Neutrophils, monocytes
Anti-CD4	Neutrophils, CD4 T lymphocytes
Anti-MPO	Neutrophils, monocytes
Anti-CD11b	Granulocytes, monocytes, some macrophages
Anti-CD11c	Granulocytes, monocytes, dendritic cells
Anti-CD11d	Macrophage subsets, T lymphocyte subsets
Other antibodies	
Anti-CD45	All leukocytes
Anti-CD11a	All leukocytes
Anti-CD34	Stem cells, early progenitor cells
Anti-class II MHC	Monocytes, B lymphocytes, T lymphocytes

Sample Preparation

Cells must be viable and in liquid suspension for flow cytometric analysis. Samples should be shipped on ice and ideally analyzed within 3 days of collection. Peripheral blood may be submitted in an EDTA collection tube. A concurrent complete blood count must be performed because a diagnosis is made based on absolute counts rather than percentages of cell subsets. Organ aspirates may be submitted in a red top tube without anticoagulant with 1 mL saline and 10% canine serum. Typically, the sample should contain enough cells to turn the solution cloudy. Cavity fluids should be submitted in an EDTA-containing tube and red top tube. These guidelines may vary slightly depending on the diagnostic laboratory and the reader should refer to the individual laboratory's submission instructions.

LYMPHOID TISSUE CYTOLOGY
Normal Cell Types

A normal lymph node aspirate contains a heterogeneous population of predominantly small mature lymphocytes, which are smaller than a neutrophil with condensed chromatin, no apparent nucleoli, and scant basophilic cytoplasm (**Fig. 2**). Intermediate lymphocytes are similar in size to a neutrophil with more dispersed chromatin, no apparent nucleoli, and expanded cytoplasm. Lymphoblasts in a normal node are slightly larger than a neutrophil with dispersed chromatin, often 1 to 2 round nucleoli and a small amount of basophilic cytoplasm. Normal peripheral blood contains

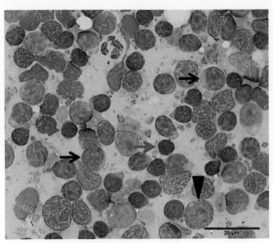

Fig. 2. Normal lymph node cytology identifying small (*red arrows*) and intermediate (*black arrows*) lymphocytes, and lymphoblasts (*arrow head*).

predominantly small mature lymphocytes, potentially with rare intermediate lymphocytes having few azurophilic granules.

Preparation and Aging Artifact

The pull-prep technique is recommended for preparation of lymph node aspirates. The goal is to obtain a sample of high cellularity where cells are able to spread out but not rupture. Quick Romanowsky-type stains tend to stain chromatin uniformly across lymphocyte subsets, making proper assessment of the chromatin difficult, and make nucleoli more prominent; therefore, stains such as the Wright-Giemsa stain are preferred.

Cytomorphology of leukocytes in the peripheral blood can change dramatically over the course of a few days, which is why fresh blood smears are crucial for proper cytology review (**Fig. 3**). Lymphocytes often swell and seem to be larger with an increased amount of cytoplasm. The chromatin may seem to be more dispersed and immature. Aging can even affect nuclear shape, creating cerebriform or clover leaf–shaped nuclei in cells that would otherwise contain round nuclei.

CYTOLOGY AND FLOW CYTOMETRY CORRELATES
Chronic Leukemias

Chronic leukemias are typically easier to classify based on morphology than other lymphoproliferative disorders because they demonstrate recognizable differentiation. Although both myeloid and lymphoid forms are seen in dogs and cats, chronic lymphocytic leukemia (CLL) is far more common than chronic myeloid leukemia.[13,14] Canine CLL generally falls into 2 major categories: B-cell CLL (B-CLL) and CD8 T-cell CLL (T-CLL). Published data suggest that T-CLL is more common than B-CLL in dogs and prognostic features have been described between and within phenotypes.[11,12,15,16] Although there can be morphologic variation within each subtype, these 2 entities generally have distinctive cytologic features.

Cases of lymphoma may have circulating neoplastic cells, but this process is distinct from CLL. For example, B cells may circulate in the peripheral blood of dogs with diffuse large B-cell lymphoma (DLBCL).[17] Currently, there are no consistent

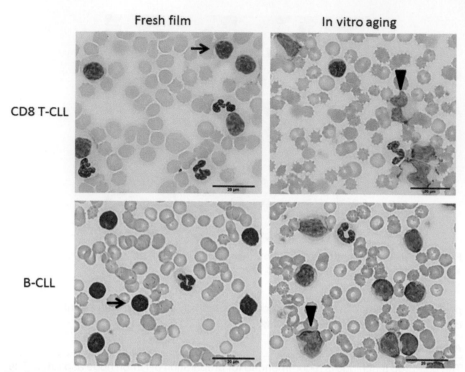

Fig. 3. Examples of aging artifact in peripheral blood. A fresh blood film (*left*) and a blood film made after in vitro aging (*right*) from the same sample in a case of CD8 T-cell leukemia (T-CLL; *top panel*) and a case of B-cell chronic lymphocytic leukemia (B-CLL; *bottom panel*) are shown. Intact cells (*arrow*) contain round nuclei, condensed chromatin and intact cytoplasm, whereas aged cells (*arrow head*) are swollen with more dispersed chromatin and variably shaped nuclei.

criteria in veterinary medicine to distinguish leukemia from lymphoma with blood infiltration, with the exception of CD34[+] acute leukemias. Differentials for persistent lymphocytosis in the dog and cat, including those of nonneoplastic origin, have been discussed previously.[18]

B-Cell Chronic Lymphocytic Leukemia

B cell chronic lymphocytic leukemia/small cell lymphoma is defined in veterinary medicine as an expansion of neoplastic small well-differentiated B cells in the peripheral blood. In human medicine, the term B-CLL/small cell lymphoma is used because patients often have lymph node involvement. Recently, 491 canine B-CLL cases were examined, which were defined as having more than 5000 lymphocytes/μL in the peripheral blood with greater than 60% of the lymphocytes being small CD21 lymphocytes.[19] As expected, peripheral cytopenias were quite rare and approximately 25% of cases had hyperglobulinemia.[19,20] Significant proportions of the dogs had peripheral lymphadenopathy, splenomegaly, and visceral lymphadenopathy supporting the use of the terminology B-CLL/small cell lymphoma. Previous studies of CLL have excluded cases with significant lymphadenopathy, which may have underestimated the reported prevalence of B-CLL.[16] Certain breeds, particularly small breed dogs, had increased odds of B-CLL, whereas large breeds such as the Golden retriever were very rarely represented.[19] B-CLL typically affects older dogs with a median age at diagnosis of 10 to 11 years.[16,19] B-CLL is frequently an incidental finding

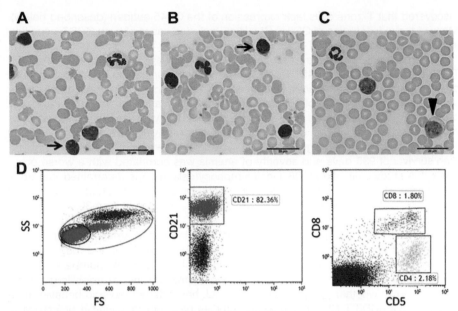

Fig. 4. Peripheral blood cytology (*A–C*) from 3 cases of canine B-cell chronic lymphocytic leukemia and characteristic flow cytometric findings (*D*). The majority of lymphocytes are small and well-differentiated (*arrow*) with rare larger more immature cells (*arrow head*). The majority of CD21 cells (*red*) fall within the small size gate, indicated by the small black circle, with small numbers of cells extending into the monocyte region.

and typically has an indolent disease course,[11] although there is some suggestion that younger age at diagnosis may be a poor prognostic indicator.[16] In a study of dogs with B-cell lymphocytosis, small cell size as determined by flow cytometry was associated with an indolent disease course and survival time of more than 1000 days.[12] A separate study evaluating outcome in 17 dogs with B-CLL determined a median survival time of 480 days.[16]

Consistent with the indolent nature of this disease, most cases of B-CLL have an expanded population of mature-appearing, small lymphocytes. These lymphocytes are typically smaller than a neutrophil, contain small, round nuclei, condensed chromatin, no apparent nucleoli, and scant rims of basophilic cytoplasm (**Fig. 4**).[13,15,16] Most cases of B-CLL contain a smaller proportion of larger, intermediate-sized lymphocytes that can be the same size or slightly larger than a neutrophil.[15,16] These cells have more dispersed chromatin and may rarely have a faint nucleolus. Flow cytometry reveals that, consistent with their morphologic appearance, the scatter properties place most cells within the area where normal small lymphocytes are located. The variable proportion of morphologically intermediate-sized cells also typically can be seen extending from this area of small cells into the area where larger cells such as monocytes typically are found.

CD8 T-Cell Chronic Lymphocytic Leukemia

What has been described as canine T-CLL is likely a heterogeneous group composed of T-zone lymphoma/leukemia and CD8 T-CLL. CD8 T-CLL cells are variably granular and often referred to as large granular lymphocyte (LGL) leukemias. This group of T-CLLs is considered the most common form of CLL in the dog, with an indolent disease course.[11,15,16] Historically, these 2 diseases were combined, until it was discovered that T-zone cells lack expression of the CD45 antigen (described below). Many of the older studies of CD8 T-CLL likely included cases of both CD8 T-zone leukemia/lymphoma and CD8 T-CLL.

Now that these 2 diseases can be differentiated easily by flow cytometry, CD8 T-CLL (defined as CD8[+] CD45[+] T cells) remains a common canine lymphoproliferative disorder and does seem to have an indolent disease course. CD8 T-CLL affects older animals with a median age of 10 years at diagnosis[16,21] and was found to affect predominantly large-breed dogs in 1 study.[21] CD8 T-CLL may be associated with splenomegaly[21] and anemia, but other cytopenias are relatively rare.[11,15,16,21] A study evaluating outcome in 19 dogs with CD8 T-CLL determined the disease has a long median survival of 930 days and severity of anemia was correlated with a worse prognosis.[16] A study evaluating CD8 T-cell lymphocytosis in dogs determined that dogs with a presenting cell count of more than 30,000 lymphocytes/μL had a significantly shorter survival time (131 days) compared with dogs with fewer than 30,000 lymphocytes/μL at presentation (1098 days).[12]

CD8 T-CLL cells are generally intermediate in size with a small round to slightly indented nucleus with clumped chromatin, no apparent nucleoli, and moderately to markedly expanded pale blue cytoplasm (**Fig. 5**).[11,15,21] Variable numbers of cells, from none to the majority, contain few to several small distinct azurophilic granules. It is not known whether nongranular CD8 T-CLL has different biologic behavior than granular (LGL) CD8 T-CLL, but previous studies have not identified a difference in outcome.[11,16] A small subset of LGL leukemias may be natural killer cell leukemias, but there is currently no way to positively identify canine natural killer cells, so we have no information about the biological behaviors of these tumors. By flow cytometry, CD8 T-CLL cells vary in FS and SS properties, with most cases falling in the region

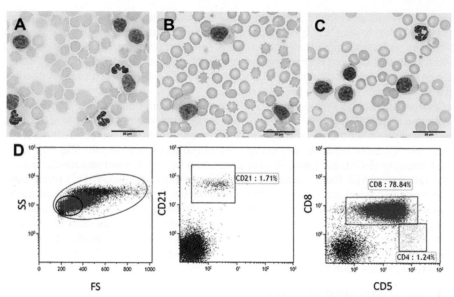

Fig. 5. Peripheral blood cytology (*A–C*) from 3 cases of canine CD8 T-cell leukemia and characteristic flow cytometry findings (*D*). The majority of lymphocytes are intermediate in size with mature chromatin and abundant pale cytoplasm. Cases vary from having few granular cells (*left*) to having predominantly granular cells (*right*). By flow cytometry, CD8[+] CD5 T cells (*magenta*) have scatter properties similar to normal small lymphocytes and monocytes. These cells express CD45.

of normal small lymphocytes and monocytes, but rare cases have abundant granular cytoplasm causing them to fall near neutrophils.

A minority of chronic *Ehrlichia canis* infections can lead to a homogeneous expansion of CD8 T cells with LGL morphology in the dog.[22,23] If there is clinical suspicion of *E canis* and a CD8 T-cell expansion of less than 30,000 cells/μL, serology testing to rule out *Ehrlichia* disease is generally recommended.

ACUTE LEUKEMIA

Acute leukemias are aggressive neoplasms of immature hematopoietic cells and may be of lymphoid origin (acute lymphocyte leukemia [ALL]), myeloid origin (acute myeloid leukemia [AML]), or undifferentiated (acute undifferentiated leukemia). They have been described based on clinical features, including circulating blast cell percentages, accompanying cytopenias and/or lack of marked peripheral lymphadenopathy, or strictly on the surface expression of the stem cell marker CD34.[12,15,24,25] The expression of the stem cell marker CD34 is an objective marker of an acute leukemia but there is evidence in people and animals that not all acute leukemias express this antigen.[25,26] In 3 studies including 8 to 25 cases, approximately 75% percent of clinically defined cases of canine acute leukemia expressed CD34.[11,13,25] Both clinical and phenotypic classification schemes have typically revealed aggressive disease progression. Studies assessing outcome determined median survival of 9 to 16 days for CD34$^+$ acute leukemia cases.[12,24] Additional difficulties arise in distinguishing acute lymphoblastic leukemia from advanced stage V lymphoma in veterinary patients, which is often based on somewhat subjective assessment of the magnitude of peripheral lymph node involvement. In people, detailed flow cytometry has allowed acute lymphoblastic lymphoma and leukemia to be classified as the same disease, arising from precursor cells in the bone marrow.[27] The morphologic assessment of blasts can vary and has not generally been codified, which, again, complicates the diagnosis of canine acute leukemias.

Because surface CD34 expression is an objective measure of an immature precursor phenotype, this review discusses the morphologic characteristics of cells from cases expressing CD34. CD34$^+$ acute leukemias consistently lack the expression of major histocompatibility complex (MHC) class II. We have reviewed the flow cytometry from 194 cases of CD34$^+$/MHC class II$^-$ leukemia and identified 3 major immunophenotypic subsets: CD5$^+$, CD14$^+$, and lineage negative/undifferentiated (manuscript in preparation). CD5$^+$ CD34$^+$ cases seem to be compatible with T-cell ALL and CD14$^+$ CD34$^+$ with AML. In addition to the CD34$^+$ cells, the AML cases consistently have a subset of CD14$^+$ cells that have lost the normal expression of MHC class II. Golden retrievers were overrepresented in the ALL group, which has been described previously,[13] and German shepherd dogs were overrepresented in the AML group. The median age at diagnosis was 8.3 years with a range of 2 to 15 years. Cytopenias were common, often affecting all 3 cell lines, and were frequently of moderate to high severity, as has been reported elsewhere.[15] Outcomes were not significantly different between flow cytometric phenotypes.

Acute leukemias have variable morphology. Cells are often intermediate to large in size with a large nucleus, dispersed chromatin, variably prominent nucleoli, and small to moderate amounts of cytoplasm (**Figs. 6** and **7**).[15] In rare cases of acute leukemia, the precursor cells can be quite small and lack overt nucleoli making the diagnosis challenging. In these cases, the presence of significant cytopenias may be the only clue that this is not a form of chronic leukemia. The morphologic overlap between acute myeloid and lymphoid leukemias can be substantial. Compared with ALL or

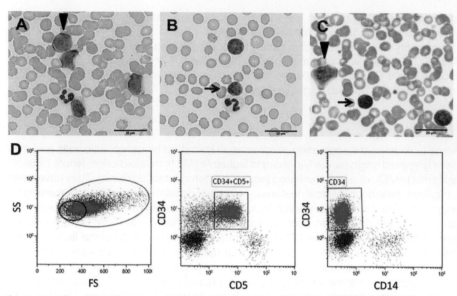

Fig. 6. Peripheral blood cytology (*A–C*) from 3 cases of canine CD5$^+$ CD34$^+$ leukemia (presumed acute lymphoid leukemia) and characteristic flow cytometry findings (*D*). Cells range from small with inconspicuous nucleoli (*arrow*) to larger with prominent nucleoli (*arrow head*). Nuclear shape varies from round to more irregular. The cells are CD34$^+$ with variable amounts of CD5 expression and generally fall within the lymphocyte and monocyte scatter zones.

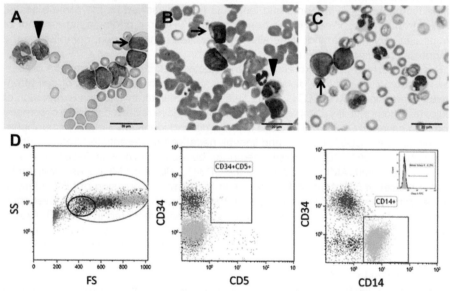

Fig. 7. Peripheral blood cytology (*A–C*) from 3 cases of canine CD14$^+$ CD34$^+$ leukemia (presumed acute myeloid leukemia) and characteristic flow cytometry findings (*D*). Cells tend to be intermediate sized to large with variably apparent nucleoli. Nuclear shape varies from round (*arrow*) to more monocytoid in appearance with indented to convoluted nuclei (*arrow head*). The cells are a mixture of smaller CD34$^+$ cells (*red*) and larger CD14$^+$/major histocompatibility complex (MHC) class II$^-$ cells (*turquoise*) by flow cytometry. The *inset* in the right panel shows the lack of MHC class II expression contrary to what is seen on normal CD14$^+$ monocytes.

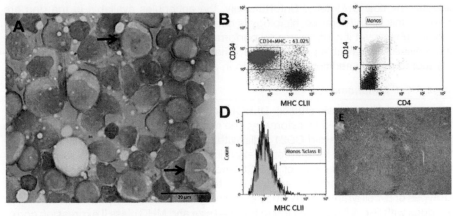

Fig. 8. Lymph node aspirate cytology results from a case of canine acute myeloid leukemia. Large, discrete cells had effaced much of the normal lymph node and some cells had a distinctive banded nuclear shape (*A, arrow*), suggestive of myeloid origin. Flow cytometry detected an expanded population of CD34$^+$/major histocompatibility complex (MHC) class II$^-$ cells (*B*) and large, CD14$^+$/MHC class II$^-$ cells (*C, D*). At necropsy, tumor cells were negative by immunohistochemical analysis for CD3 and Pax5 and were strongly positive for the myeloid marker CD18 (*E*).

acute undifferentiated leukemia, AML cells may have a more irregularly shaped nucleus, lower nuclear:cytoplasmic ratio, variably sized vacuoles, and/or pink or purple granules. AML cases often progress toward some degree of monocytoid appearance, whereas ALL cases often maintain round to ovoid nuclei and scant amounts of cytoplasm.

Acute leukemias can infiltrate lymph nodes and other solid tissues such as spleen, liver, and kidney (**Fig. 8**). When large immature round cells are seen in tissues and they do not have the morphology of the classic lymphoma subsets described, flow cytometry is a useful tool for further characterization. When acute leukemia cells infiltrate tissues, they often do not efface the normal tissue and there may still be normal residual lymph node, but flow cytometry can identify a population of CD34$^+$/MHC class II$^-$ cells allowing for diagnosis.

LYMPHOMA

The most common form of lymphoma in dogs is multicentric lymphoma, affecting peripheral lymph nodes.[28,29] B-cell lymphoma is more common than T-cell lymphoma. Several histologic forms of B-cell lymphoma have been identified in the dog and the subset DLBCL is by far the most common.[28–30] The major forms of T-cell lymphoma in the dog are aggressive peripheral T-cell lymphoma and T-zone lymphoma. Aggressive peripheral T-cell lymphoma includes the subsets peripheral T-cell lymphoma not otherwise specified and lymphoblastic T-cell lymphoma.[31,32] As mentioned, cytology is a reliable and sensitive diagnostic technique to reach the diagnosis of lymphoma in most canine cases. This is largely owing to the diffuse nature and larger lymphocyte size of the more common forms of canine lymphoma allowing the detection of lymph node effacement by the proliferating neoplastic lymphocytes. The common forms of canine lymphoma have distinguishing cytologic features, although the morphology of less common subtypes is less well-known. In human medicine, the majority of lymphoma subtypes can be defined based on unique immunophenotypic features, detected by flow cytometry. Unfortunately, the antibodies available in the dog are limited at this time. Therefore, histology is needed for definitive diagnosis of most lymphoma subsets yet it is uncommonly performed in clinical situations. Flow cytometry can provide very valuable prognostic information and has emerged as a complimentary tool to provide additional information in a noninvasive fashion.

Large B-Cell Lymphoma

In a number of large-scale studies, DLBCL accounted for the majority of canine lymphoma cases.[28,29,33] By flow cytometry, the majority of cases of B-cell lymphoma are composed of medium-sized CD21 cells with variable, although generally high, MHC class II expression. We have recently examined the flow cytometry findings from 37 histologically confirmed cases of DLBCL and found this to be the consistent phenotype.[34] Further studies are needed to correlate flow cytometric findings with histologic subtypes of B-cell lymphoma. A study examining immunophenotype characteristics in 160 dogs with B-cell lymphoma found that cell size and MHC class II expression correlated with a worse prognosis.[35,36] Dogs with medium-sized cells and high MHC class II expression had a median survival of 330 days whereas large-sized cells and low MHC class II expression were poor prognostic indicators.[35] Rarely, these B-cell lymphoma cases may coexpress CD34 while retaining MHC class II expression, but this aberrant expression does not seem to affect the outcome and these cases should not be misdiagnosed as acute leukemias.[35] This study demonstrates that there is some heterogeneity among large B-cell lymphomas, and flow cytometry can be useful in predicting outcome.

Cytologically, the lymphocytes in these large B-cell lymphomas can be variable in size, but are often 1 to 1.5 times the size of a neutrophil with a large round nucleus, dispersed immature chromatin, often 1 to 2 large round prominent nucleoli, and a small amount of deeply basophilic cytoplasm (**Fig. 9**).[37,38] Cytoplasm may contain small numbers of small clear punctate vacuoles and mitotic figures are common. By flow cytometry, the majority of cases have a dramatic expansion of medium-sized CD21 cells. Smaller numbers of cases have large-sized cells by flow cytometry.

CD4 T-Cell Lymphoma

In our experience, CD4 T-cell lymphoma is the most common form of multicentric T-cell lymphoma, which is supported by 2 small case series of canine lymphoma.[39,40] There is a breed predilection for Boxers and Golden retrievers.[31,32,41] The CD4 phenotype is associated with an aggressive clinical course and increased incidence of hypercalcemia and mediastinal masses.[31,32,41–44] In a study examining 61 cases of CD4 T-cell lymphoma, the median survival was 159 days.[31] Among the 15 biopsies evaluated in this study, 10 were histologically classified as peripheral T-cell lymphoma not otherwise specified and 5 as lymphoblastic T cell lymphoma. There were no clinical or flow cytometric differences between the 2 histologic subsets. By flow cytometry, neoplastic cells have uniform expression of CD3 and CD45, low levels of MHC class II, and variable expression of CD5. In 1 study, CD5 expression had a small impact on overall survival and flow cytometric cell size had a moderate impact on the progression-free interval and overall survival.[31]

Lymphocytes are intermediately sized, similar in size to a neutrophil with a round to indented nucleus, dispersed to dusty chromatin, no apparent nucleoli, and moderately expanded pale blue cytoplasm, without granules or vacuoles (**Fig. 10**).[37,38] Cytologically, CD4 T-cell lymphoma may seem less aggressive because cells generally lack nucleoli, but this type of lymphoma has a worse overall prognosis than DLBCL, which has prominent nucleoli.

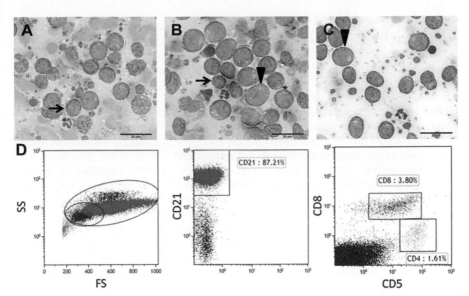

Fig. 9. Lymph node aspirate cytology (*A–C*) from 3 cases of canine large B-cell lymphoma and characteristic flow cytometry findings (*D*). Basophilic lymphoblasts with a round nucleus and prominent nucleoli vary in size from the same size as a neutrophil (*arrow*) to 1.5 to 2 times the size of a neutrophil (*arrow head*). By flow cytometry, CD21 cells comprise the vast majority of the cells (*red*) and are medium to large in size. Major histocompatibility complex class II expression is typically high with smaller numbers of cases having low level expression (not shown).

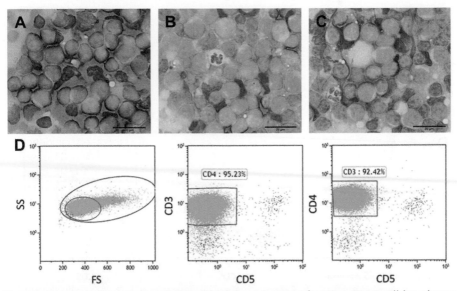

Fig. 10. Lymph node aspirate cytology (*A–C*) from 3 cases of canine CD4 T-cell lymphoma and characteristic flow cytometry findings (*D*). Lymphocytes have round to indented nuclei, dispersed chromatin, and expanded pale staining cytoplasm. Nucleoli are typically not visible in most cells. CD4 T cells (*green*) are generally intermediate sized with some overlap with normal lymphocytes. A subset of these cases, as shown here in the center and right panels, have lost the expression of the pan–T-cell antigen CD5.

T-Zone Disease (Lymphoma/Leukemia)

T-zone lymphoma is a subtype of peripheral T-cell lymphoma with an indolent disease course. Recently, T-zone T cells were discovered to lack expression of the pan-leukocyte CD45 antigen.[45,46] This unique immunophenotype allows for the diagnosis of T-zone lymphoma by flow cytometry, rather than the more invasive method of biopsy and histology. These cells may express surface CD4, CD8, neither CD4 nor CD8, or very rarely both antigens. T-zone cells often express CD21. Lymphocytosis is associated very commonly with T-zone lymphoma,[45,47,48] which is why the term T-zone disease (lymphoma/leukemia) may be used. The simple presence of circulating T-zone cells in the peripheral blood is not associated with a worse prognosis than those cases without lymphocytosis.[47] T-zone disease is often identified as an incidental finding of lymphocytosis or lymphadenopathy.[49] The estimated prevalence of T-zone disease is 3% to 13% of all canine lymphomas,[28,34] and the overall median survival times have ranged from 21.2 to 33.5 months.[45,47,48] T-zone disease affects older dogs, with a median age at diagnosis of 10 years.[45,48] There is a strong breed predilection, with 40% of all cases being Golden retrievers.[45] It is important to differentiate T-zone disease from other forms of T-cell lymphoma, because T-zone disease has an indolent disease course and does not seem to require aggressive chemotherapy treatment.[47]

In the peripheral blood, T-zone cells are typically similar in size to a neutrophil with a round centrally located nucleus, coarse chromatin, rarely 1 small faint nucleolus, and a full rim of mildly to moderately expanded pale blue cytoplasm (**Fig. 11**).[50] There may be overlap in morphology between some T-zone cells and CD8 T-CLL cells in the blood, but generally CD8 T-CLL have more abundant irregularly shaped cytoplasm.

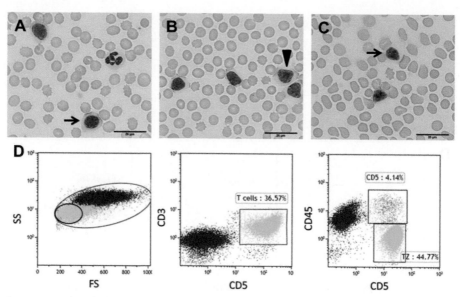

Fig. 11. Peripheral blood cytology (*A–C*) from 3 cases of canine T-zone disease and characteristic flow cytometry findings (*D*). T-zone cells with evenly distributed, mildly expanded cytoplasm are indicated with the arrow. More irregular T-zone cells with morphology similar to CD8 T-cell chronic lymphocytic leukemia are indicated with the *arrowhead*. The flow cytometry demonstrates small to intermediate-sized CD3+/CD5+ T cells (*turquoise*) with the characteristic loss of CD45 expression (*right*).

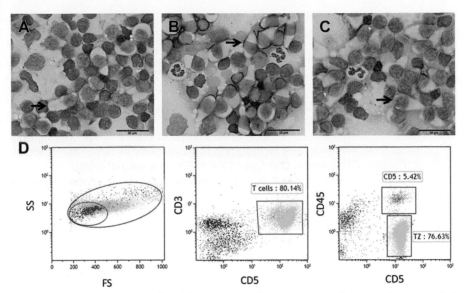

Fig. 12. Lymph node cytology (*A–C*) from 3 cases of canine T-zone disease and characteristic flow cytometry findings (*D*). T-zone cells vary in number from smaller numbers (*left*) to many (*right*). These cells have the classic expanded, pale cytoplasm, which often forms the mirror-handle appearance described in the text (*arrows*). T-zone cells (*turquoise*) express the pan–T-cell markers CD3 and CD5, lack CD45 expression and are small to intermediate in size.

In lymph node aspirates, T-zone cells are intermediate in size with a small round eccentrically placed nucleus, coarse chromatin, and rarely a faint nucleolus. There is often an asymmetric expansion of pale cytoplasm, forming a wide-based, mirror-handle appearance (**Fig. 12**).[28,50] These mirror-handle structures can be created artificially in non–T-zone lymphocytes owing to preparation artifact, but then the structures generally are not evenly distributed on the slide and have a narrow base, as opposed to the wider base in T-zone cells. Although T-zone cells have a small, relatively mature-appearing nucleus, the overall cell size is intermediate owing to the expanded cytoplasm and cells fall between small lymphocytes and monocytes by flow cytometry.

SUMMARY

Cytology is a useful diagnostic tool to establish the initial diagnosis of lymphoma and leukemia, and cytologic features may be present that suggest a particular subtype of disease. Flow cytometry remains a vital, noninvasive tool to confirm cytologic impressions and can provide valuable information in formulating a prognosis.

REFERENCES

1. Sato H, Fujino Y, Chino J, et al. Prognostic analyses on anatomical and morphological classification of feline lymphoma. J Vet Med Sci 2014;76(6): 807–11.
2. Valentini F, Tasca S, Gavazza A, et al. Use of CD9 and CD61 for the characterization of AML-M7 by flow cytometry in a dog. Vet Comp Oncol 2012;10(4): 312–8.

3. Wilkerson MJ. Principles and applications of flow cytometry and cell sorting in companion animal medicine. Vet Clin North Am Small Anim Pract 2012;42(1): 53–71.

4. Comazzi S, Gelain ME. Use of flow cytometric immunophenotyping to refine the cytological diagnosis of canine lymphoma. Vet J 2011;188(2):149–55.

5. Avery AC. Immunophenotyping and determination of clonality. In: Weiss DJ, Wardrop KJ, editors. Schalm's veterinary hematology. 6th edition. Hoboken (NJ): Wiley-Blackwell; 2011. p. 1133–206.

6. Comazzi S, Avery PR, Garden OA, et al. European canine lymphoma network consensus recommendations for reporting flow cytometry in canine hematopoietic neoplasms. Cytometry B Clin Cytom 2016. [Epub ahead of print].

7. Faldyna M, Levá L, Knötigová P, et al. Lymphocyte subsets in peripheral blood of dogs - a flow cytometric study. Vet Immunol Immunopathol 2001;82(1–2):23–37.

8. Watabe A, Fukumoto S, Komatsu T, et al. Alterations of lymphocyte subpopulations in healthy dogs with aging and in dogs with cancer. Vet Immunol Immunopathol 2011;142(3–4):189–200.

9. Faldyna M, Sinkora J, Knotigova P, et al. Lymphatic organ development in dogs: major lymphocyte subsets and activity. Vet Immunol Immunopathol 2005; 104(3–4):239–47.

10. Wilkerson MJ, Dolce K, Koopman T, et al. Lineage differentiation of canine lymphoma/leukemias and aberrant expression of CD molecules. Vet Immunol Immunopathol 2005;106(3–4):179–96.

11. Vernau W, Moore PF. An immunophenotypic study of canine leukemias and preliminary assessment of clonality by polymerase chain reaction. Vet Immunol Immunopathol 1999;69(2–4):145–64.

12. Williams MJ, Avery AC, Lana SE, et al. Canine Lymphoproliferative disease characterized by lymphocytosis: immunophenotypic markers of prognosis. J Vet Intern Med 2008;22(3):596–601.

13. Adam F, Villiers E, Watson S, et al. Clinical pathological and epidemiological assessment of morphologically and immunologically confirmed canine leukaemia. Vet Comp Oncol 2009;7(3):181–95.

14. Workman HC, Vernau W. Chronic lymphocytic leukemia in dogs and cats: the veterinary perspective. Vet Clin North Am Small Anim Pract 2003;33(6):1379–99.

15. Tasca S, Carli E, Caldin M, et al. Hematologic abnormalities and flow cytometric immunophenotyping results in dogs with hematopoietic neoplasia: 210 cases (2002-2006). Vet Clin Pathol 2009;38(1):2–12.

16. Comazzi S, Gelain ME, Martini V, et al. Immunophenotype predicts survival time in dogs with chronic lymphocytic leukemia. J Vet Intern Med 2011;25(1):100–6.

17. Martini V, Melzi E, Comazzi S, et al. Peripheral blood abnormalities and bone marrow infiltration in canine large B-cell lymphoma: Is there a link? Vet Comp Oncol 2015;13(2):117–23.

18. Avery AC, Avery PR. Determining the significance of persistent lymphocytosis. Vet Clin North Am Small Anim Pract 2007;37(2):267–82.

19. Bromberek JL, Rout ED, Agnew MR, et al. Breed distribution and clinical characteristics of B cell chronic lymphocytic leukemia in dogs. J Vet Intern Med 2016;30: 215–22.

20. Leifer C, Matus R. Chronic lymphocytic leukemia in the dog: 22 cases (1974-1984). J Am Vet Med Assoc 1986;189(2):214–7.

21. McDonough SP, Moore PF. Clinical, hematologic, and immunophenotypic characterization of canine large granular lymphocytosis. Vet Pathol 2000;37(6):637–46.

22. Heeb HL, Wilkerson MJ, Chun R, et al. Large granular lymphocytosis, lymphocyte subset inversion, thrombocytopenia, dysproteinemia, and positive Ehrlichia serology in a dog. J Am Anim Hosp Assoc 2003;39(4):379–84.

23. Weiser MG, Thrall MA, Fulton R, et al. Granular lymphocytosis and hyperproteinemia in dogs with chronic ehrlichiosis. J Am Anim Hosp Assoc 1991;27:84–8.

24. Novacco M, Comazzi S, Marconato L, et al. Prognostic factors in canine acute leukaemias: A retrospective study. Vet Comp Oncol 2015. [Epub ahead of print].

25. Villiers E, Baines S, Law AM, et al. Identification of acute myeloid leukemia in dogs using flow cytometry with myeloperoxidase, MAC387, and a canine neutrophil-specific antibody. Vet Clin Pathol 2006;35(1):55–71.

26. Sperling C, Buchner T, Creutzig U, et al. Clinical, morphologic, cytogenetic and prognostic implications of CD34 expression in childhood and adult de novo AML. Leuk Lymphoma 1995;17(5–6):417–26.

27. Han X, Bueso-Ramos CE. Precursor T-cell acute lymphoblastic leukemia/lymphoblastic lymphoma and acute biphenotypic leukemias. Am J Clin Pathol 2007; 127(4):528–44.

28. Ponce F, Marchal T, Magnol JP, et al. A morphological study of 608 cases of canine malignant lymphoma in France with a focus on comparative similarities between canine and human lymphoma morphology. Vet Pathol 2010;47:414–33.

29. Vezzali E, Parodi AL, Marcato PS, et al. Histopathologic classification of 171 cases of canine and feline non-Hodgkin lymphoma according to the WHO. Vet Comp Oncol 2010;8(1):38–49.

30. Valli VE, Kass PH, San Myint M, et al. Canine lymphomas: association of classification type, disease stage, tumor subtype, mitotic rate, and treatment with survival. Vet Pathol 2013;50(5):738–48.

31. Avery PR, Burton J, Bromberek JL, et al. Flow cytometric characterization and clinical outcome of CD4+ T-cell lymphoma in dogs: 67 cases. J Vet Intern Med 2014;28(2):538–46.

32. Lurie DM, Milner RJ, Suter SE, et al. Immunophenotypic and cytomorphologic subclassification of T-cell lymphoma in the boxer breed. Vet Immunol Immunopathol 2008;125(1–2):102–10.

33. Valli VE, San Myint M, Barthel A, et al. Classification of canine malignant lymphomas according to the World Health Organization criteria. Vet Pathol 2011; 48(1):198–211.

34. Curran KM, Schaffer PA, Frank CB, et al. BCL2 and MYC are expressed at high levels in canine diffuse large B cell lymphoma but are not predictive for outcome in dogs treated with CHOP chemotherapy. Vet Comp Onc 2016. in press.

35. Rao S, Lana S, Eickhoff J, et al. Class II major histocompatibility complex expression and cell size independently predict survival in canine B-cell lymphoma. J Vet Intern Med 2011;25(5):1097–105.

36. Pinheiro D, Chang YM, Bryant H, et al. Dissecting the regulatory microenvironment of a large animal model of non-Hodgkin lymphoma: evidence of a negative prognostic impact of FOXP3+ T cells in canine B cell lymphoma. PLoS One 2014; 9(8):e105027.

37. Zandvliet M. Canine lymphoma: a review. Vet Q 2016;36(2):76–104.

38. Ponce F, Magnol JP, Ledieu D, et al. Prognostic significance of morphological subtypes in canine malignant lymphomas during chemotherapy. Vet J 2004; 167(2):158–66.

39. Culmsee K, Simon D, Mischke R, et al. Possibilities of flow cytometric analysis for immunophenotypic characterization of canine lymphoma. J Vet Med A Physiol Pathol Clin Med 2001;48(4):199–206.

40. Gelain ME, Mazzilli M, Riondato F, et al. Aberrant phenotypes and quantitative antigen expression in different subtypes of canine lymphoma by flow cytometry. Vet Immunol Immunopathol 2008;121(3–4):179–88.
41. Lurie DM, Lucroy MD, Griffey SM, et al. T-cell-derived malignant lymphoma in the boxer breed. Vet Comp Oncol 2004;2(3):171–5.
42. Ruslander DA, Gebhard DH, Tompkins MB, et al. Immunophenotypic characterization of canine lymphoproliferative disorders. In Vivo 1997;11:169–72.
43. Rebhun RB, Kent MS, Borrofka SA, et al. CHOP chemotherapy for the treatment of canine multicentric T-cell lymphoma. Vet Comp Oncol 2011;9(1):38–44.
44. Brodsky EM, Maudlin GN, Lachowicz JL, et al. Asparaginase and MOPP treatment of dogs with lymphoma. J Vet Intern Med 2009;23(3):578–84.
45. Seelig DM, Avery P, Webb T, et al. Canine T-zone lymphoma: unique immunophenotypic features, outcome, and population characteristics. J Vet Intern Med 2014; 28(3):878–86.
46. Martini V, Poggi A, Riondato F, et al. Flow-cytometric detection of phenotypic aberrancies in canine small clear cell lymphoma. Vet Comp Oncol 2013;13(3): 281–7.
47. Flood-Knapik KE, Durham AC, Gregor TP, et al. Clinical, histopathological and immunohistochemical characterization of canine indolent lymphoma. Vet Comp Oncol 2013;11(4):272–86.
48. Martini V, Marconato L, Poggi A, et al. Canine small clear cell/T-zone lymphoma: clinical presentation and outcome in a retrospective case series. Vet Comp Oncol 2015. [Epub ahead of print].
49. Valli VE, Vernau W, de Lorimier LP, et al. Canine indolent nodular lymphoma. Vet Pathol 2006;43(3):241–56.
50. Mizutani N, Goto-Koshino Y, Takahashi M, et al. Clinical and histopathological evaluation of 16 dogs with T-zone lymphoma. J Vet Med Sci 2016. [Epub ahead of print].

Cytology of Bone

Anne M. Barger, DVM, MS

KEYWORDS

- Bone • Cytology • Osteosarcoma • Osteomyelitis

KEY POINTS

- Aspiration of bone lesions can be rewarding and is beneficial in differentiating inflammatory from neoplastic processes.
- Cytology is a component of the diagnostic process and should be combined with signalment, history and radiographic findings to come to a final diagnosis.
- Different techniques and imaging modalities are available to assist with successful aspiration of lesions.

INTRODUCTION

Fine-needle aspiration of bone lesions is becoming a more common diagnostic technique in human and veterinary medicine. Indications for aspiration include evidence of cortical lysis or periosteal proliferation. Occasionally, these lesions also consist of a palpable soft tissue mass. Imaging is necessary to confirm the presence of boney involvement.

CYTOLOGY VERSUS HISTOPATHOLOGY

Cytology has some significant advantages but is not without its limitations. Cytology is less expensive than biopsy on multiple levels. The biopsy procedure itself is more expensive because it requires specific equipment and sedation or general anesthesia. The biopsy testing performed by the laboratory is more expensive because significant tissue processing is involved. The turn-around time for cytology is quicker, particularly with bone samples, because the tissue preparation of bone often requires a decalcification process, which can take several days depending on the size of the tissue submitted. Biopsies are more invasive with larger pieces of tissue being removed compared with aspirates; therefore, there is a greater risk for complications such as pathologic fracture and wound infection. There are also significant limitations to cytology. Bone can be challenging to aspirate, so there is a risk of low cellularity samples or aspiration of reactive bone instead of the primary lesion. The level of diagnosis may not be as specific as can be obtained with biopsy. For instance, cytology may

The author has nothing to disclose.
Pathobiology Department, University of Illinois, 1008 Hazelwood Drive, Urbana, IL 61802, USA
E-mail address: abarger@illinois.edu

Vet Clin Small Anim 47 (2017) 71–84
http://dx.doi.org/10.1016/j.cvsm.2016.07.005
0195-5616/17/© 2016 Elsevier Inc. All rights reserved.

result in a diagnosis of sarcoma, whereas biopsy may be able to provide a more-specific diagnosis, including the type of tumor, based on the architecture of the tissue and the constitution of the background matrix. Often the amount of tissue removed with a biopsy is small enough to limit these advantages, however. Several studies compared the accuracy of cytology with histopathology as the gold standard. In human pathology, cytology was correctly able to identify malignant neoplasia in soft-tissue, musculoskeletal tumors, and bone tumors 98% of the time.[1] In a second study focused on only bone tumors, cytology findings agreed with those of histopathology 80% of the time.[2] Both benign and malignant tumors were evaluated in this study. In a study specifically focused on osteosarcoma, cytology correctly diagnosed osteosarcoma in 83% of cases with 17% of cases considered nondiagnostic with cytology.[3] In dogs, cytology was able to differentiate sarcoma from benign lesions with 97% sensitivity and 97% accuracy.[4] In a retrospective study of histologically confirmed osteosarcoma, cytology had 70% partial or full agreement with histopathology,[5] suggesting that cytology is a worthwhile diagnostic tool in the diagnosis of bone neoplasia (**Table 1**).

ASPIRATION OF BONE

There are multiple techniques available for bone aspiration, and the equipment necessary is limited and inexpensive. A range of needle sizes can be used depending on the level of lysis in the lesion. In highly lytic lesions, a 22-gauge needle can be used with success.[6] Generally, however, larger-gauge needles such as 16 or 18 gauge are more commonly used. True fine-needle aspiration, with a needle attached to a 6- or a 12-mL syringe is effective. The fenestration technique, with a needle only or a needle attached to a syringe with the plunger extended, is also a useful technique (**Fig. 1**). Neoplastic and inflammatory bone lesions often have a proliferative response of healthy osteoblasts, attempting to stabilize the bone. Therefore, it is important to aspirate bone masses or lytic lesions in the center of the lesion rather than at the periphery. This procedure can generally be done using radiographs and anatomic landmarks to identify the best area. If additional imaging is needed, ultrasound guidance and computed tomography may be beneficial. In one study, using ultrasound guidance, a diagnostic sample was obtained in 32 of 36 cases.[4] Computed tomography guidance was also evaluated for bone aspiration; however, this was done in a postmortem

---

Table 1
Advantages and disadvantages of cytology versus histopathology

	Cytology	Histopathology
Expense and equipment	Inexpensive, minimal equipment needed	More expensive than cytology, specialized equipment needed
Effect on patient	Minimally invasive, minimal risk of complications, sedation may not be required	Sedation required, risk of possible infection or fracture at biopsy site
Diagnostic quality	Can be excellent but risk of low cellular sample or aspiration of reactive bone rather than primary lesion	Can be a very specific diagnosis, but if sample size is too small, may not be enough architecture or cellular product for specific diagnosis
Turnaround time	Can be quick, within 24 h	Decalcification of sample may be required, which could delay results by 1–2 d

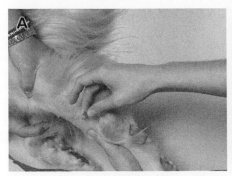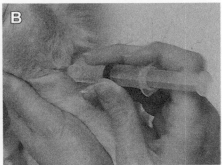

Fig. 1. (*A*) Aspiration of a lytic bone lesion with soft swelling using the fenestration technique with the needle only. (*B*) Aspiration of the same mass as in **Fig. 1**A, also using the fenestration technique with the syringe attached, plunger extended.

study and may not be of any added value for ante mortem samples.[7] Different aspiration methods have also been studied. A method of core aspiration cytology, using a 16-gauge bone marrow biopsy needle, which theoretically had a better chance of penetrating the bone cortex, has been used in dogs.[8] This technique, however, did not have any advantage over standard fine-needle aspiration.

BONE CYTOLOGY

Healthy bone consists of mineralized tissue (osteoid) with small cells, osteocytes, housed in small lacunae within the osteoid. Osteoblasts exist on the bone surface and produce osteoid and initiate the mineralization of the matrix.[9] Osteoclasts are multinucleated cells responsible for resorption of bone. Osteoclasts and osteoblasts combine their efforts for effective bone remodeling. Finally, the surface of the bone is covered by fibrous connective tissue called periosteum. The cells that can be seen in healthy bone include osteoblasts, osteoclasts, chondrocytes, and periosteal cells. Because of the mineralized matrix, it is difficult to aspirate intact, healthy, bone. The sample is often of low cellularity and may only consist of red blood cells and low numbers of the constituents of bone. Osteoblasts are round and often plasmacytoid in appearance. They have a small, eccentrically placed nucleus. The chromatin pattern is finely stippled. These cells often have a perinuclear clearing that in human medicine is referred to as a *perinuclear Hof*[10] (**Fig. 2**). Osteoclasts are multinucleated cells containing multiple uniform nuclei. The cytoplasm is basophilic, usually containing a light dusting of eosinophilic granules (**Fig. 3**). Chondrocytes are usually seen in bone aspirates taken near the joint. These cells are small and round and are often associated with small fragments of cartilage. Periosteal cells are thin mesenchymal cells with long cytoplasmic projections and long narrow nuclei (**Fig. 4**).

REACTIVE BONE

The term *reactive bone* refers to a nonneoplastic proliferation of osteoblasts in response to damage to the bone. It can be seen in response to trauma, inflammation, and neoplasia. Aspirates from these areas can be highly cellular. The cells consist primarily of reactive osteoblasts. These cells are round with deeply basophilic cytoplasm caused by the abundant rough endoplasmic reticulum and mitochondria.[9] These cells will also have a prominent Golgi apparatus, which appears cytologically as a prominent perinuclear clearing (**Fig. 5**). Compared with nonreactive osteoblasts, reactive

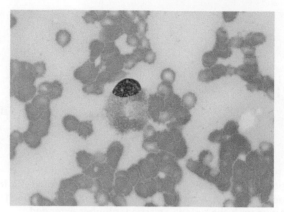

Fig. 2. Cytology from a lytic bone lesion in a dog, pictured is a cytologically unremarkable osteoblast. Not the eccentrically placed nucleus and prominent perinuclear clearing (Wright-Giemsa stain, original magnification, x1000).

osteoblasts can exhibit moderate anisocytosis and anisokaryosis and have prominent nucleoli. The nuclear/cytoplasmic ratio is still low, because these cells have small nuclei and abundant amounts of cytoplasm.[10] Because these reactive osteoblasts exhibit some cellular atypia, it is critical not to confuse them with neoplastic osteoblasts (**Fig. 6**).

OSTEOMYELITIS

Osteomyelitis indicates inflammation of the bone and can result secondary to infection with bacterial, fungal or, less commonly, protozoal organisms. Bacterial osteomyelitis often occurs secondary to an inciting injury like a bite wound, open fracture, foreign body, or postsurgical infection. Although primary hematogenous infection is possible, it is uncommon. *Actinomyces* sp and *Nocardia* sp organisms are reported to cause bacterial osteomyelitis. Cytologically, these infections are usually suppurative and

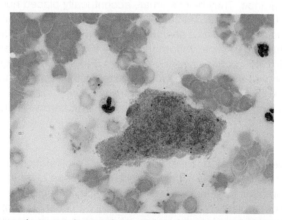

Fig. 3. Aspirate from the same dog as **Fig. 2**. Pictured is an osteoclast. These cells are multinucleated and often contain deeply eosinophilic granular material within the cytoplasm (Wright-Giemsa stain, original magnification, x1000).

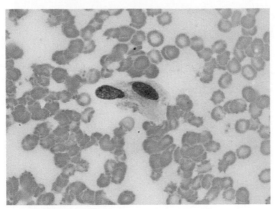

Fig. 4. Aspirate from a proliferative lesion in a dog. The sample is of low cellularity. Only rare thin mesenchymal cells are identified, consistent with periosteal cells (Wright-Giemsa stain, original magnification, x1000).

predominated by neutrophils, which are often degenerate.[11] Intralesional bacteria are identified regularly. Pyogranulomatous inflammation is also recognized with nocardial osteomyelitis.[12]

Fungal organisms known to cause osteomyelitis include *Blastomyces dermatitidis*, *Histoplasma capsulatum*, *Cryptococcus* sp, *Coccidioides* sp, *Aspergillus* sp, and *Geomyces* sp.[13] Cytologically, the samples are generally highly cellular and consist of a mixed inflammatory response predominated by neutrophils with lesser numbers of epithelioid macrophages and multinucleated giant cells. Although fungal osteomyelitis typically elicits a pyogranulomatous inflammatory response, occasionally, infection with fungal organisms can result in suppurative osteomyelitis particularly with *B dermatitidis*.[14] For most of these organisms, the yeast form of the fungus is identified in aspirates, but hyphae can also be seen (**Fig. 7**). Each organism has distinct morphologic features. *B dermatitidis* yeasts range in size from 5 to 20 µm. These yeasts are

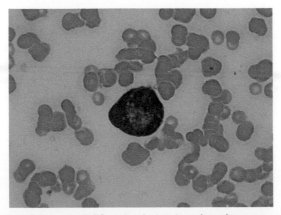

Fig. 5. Aspirate from a lytic and proliferative lesion in a dog, the mass was aspirated at the periphery. Pictured is a typical reactive osteoblast with deeply basophilic cytoplasm, a small round nucleus with a prominent Golgi apparatus (Wright-Giemsa stain, original magnification, x1000).

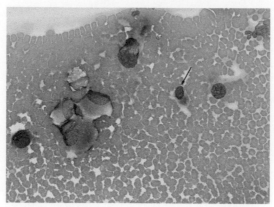

Fig. 6. Aspirate from an area of lysis in the distal radius from a dog. Overall, the sample consisted of a mixture of neoplastic osteoblasts and few reactive osteoblasts. The arrow indicates a likely osteoblast (Wright-Giemsa stain, original magnification, x500).

round with a double-contoured wall and characteristic broad-based budding (**Fig. 8**). *H capsulatum* yeasts are much smaller (2–4 μm) with a thin capsule and crescent shaped to round eosinophilic nuclei. These organisms are often observed within the cytoplasm of macrophages but can also be identified extracellularly (**Fig. 9**). *Cryptococcus* sp is diagnosed more frequently in cats than dogs, although cryptococcal osteomyelitis has been reported in dogs.[15] The organisms are round and vary greatly in size (3–10 μm). In the tissue, the organisms have a thick mucinous, nonstaining capsule. In the absence of a capsule, however, these organisms can be difficult to distinguish from blastomycosis. Therefore, the presence of the characteristic narrow-based budding is useful. *Coccidioides immitis* organisms are quite large (10–100 μm). They are round and contain high numbers of endospores (**Fig. 10**).

Rarely, protozoal organisms such as *Hepatozoon* sp are reported to cause osteomyelitis.[16] Lesions can contain meronts filled with multiple micromerozoites.

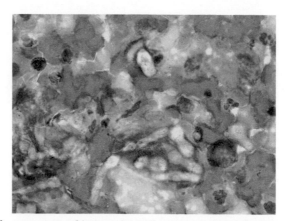

Fig. 7. Aspirate from an area of lysis and proliferation in the distal femur from a German shepherd dog. Many nonstaining fungal hyphae are observed. Culture and polymerase chain reaction confirmed *Aspergillus fumigatus* (Wright-Giemsa stain, original magnification, x1000).

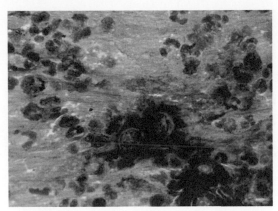

Fig. 8. Aspirate from a small lytic lesion in the carpus of a dog. The sample was cellular, a mixed inflammatory population is observed with low numbers of fungal yeast consistent with *B dermatitidis* (Wright-Giemsa stain, original magnification, x1000).

NEOPLASIA

Tumors associated with bone lysis or proliferation are categorized as primary bone tumors (tumors that arise from cells associated with bone), tumors of bone marrow origin, or metastatic bone neoplasms. Several tissues are involved in the formation of healthy bone; therefore, several tumors are considered primary bone tumors. These tumors include fibrosarcoma, osteosarcoma, chondrosarcoma, synovial cell sarcoma, histiocytic sarcoma, and hemangiosarcoma. Many of these tumors appear cytologically similar with a few distinguishing features. Generally, the aspirates are much more cellular than an aspirate of healthy or even reactive bone because of the lysis of the matrix and the disorganized proliferation of neoplastic cells. The cells vary in shape from round to spindle shaped with basophilic cytoplasm and round to oval nuclei. Obvious criteria of malignancy are easily recognized. Often, cytology can give a diagnosis of sarcoma with a more specific diagnosis requiring special staining. Some features allow ranking of the previously mentioned primary bone tumors higher

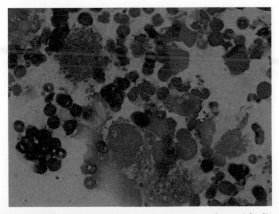

Fig. 9. Aspirate from one of multiple lytic bone lesions in a dog with diarrhea. Many extracellular and intracellular fungal yeast organisms consistent with *H capsulatum* are identified (Wright-Giemsa stain, original magnification, x1000).

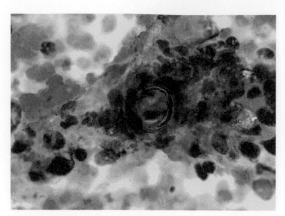

Fig. 10. Aspirate of a scapular mass from a dog that had recently traveled to Arizona. Rare large yeast organisms consistent with *C immitis* are observed (Wright-Giemsa stain, original magnification, x1000).

in the differential list; these include location of the lesion, radiographic appearance, and breed in addition to specific cytologic features.

Chondrosarcomas can have abundant amounts of eosinophilic matrix in the background and vibrantly staining eosinophilic material within the cytoplasm[17] (**Fig. 11**). Location can also assist in the diagnosis of chondrosarcoma. These tumors are more likely to occur in the rib and maxilla, although these tumors can occur in the long bones as well.[18] Fibrosarcoma is more likely to consist of spindle-shaped cells when compared with osteosarcoma and chondrosarcoma.

Osteosarcoma cells are often described as plasmacytoid because they can be round and have an eccentrically placed nucleus and sometimes a perinuclear clearing (**Fig. 12**). Common features of osteosarcoma include marked criteria of malignancy with decreased nuclear/cytoplasmic ratio, eosinophilic granulation of the cytoplasm, and presence of mitotic figures, all good indicators of malignancy.[19] Erythrophagia has also been noted in osteosarcoma but is also a feature of other sarcomas as well, including hemangiosarcoma and histiocytic sarcoma.[20] Aspirates of suspected

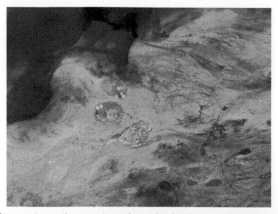

Fig. 11. Aspirate from a lytic rib mass in a dog. The background is filled with deeply eosinophilic matrix, making it difficult to identify the nucleated cell population. This aspirate is typical of a chondrosarcoma (Wright-Giemsa stain, original magnification, x500).

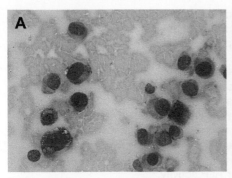
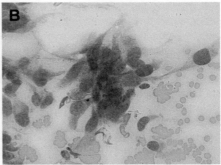

Fig. 12. (*A*) Cytology from a proximal humerus mass in a Rottweiler. The cells are round and have a typical plasmacytoid appearance consistent with osteosarcoma. Erythrophagia is also noted in many cells (Wright-Giemsa stain, original magnification, x500). (*B*) Cytology from a jaw mass in a dog. The cells are markedly spindle shaped, but cells were positive for ALP activity, and osteosarcoma was confirmed with histopathology (Wright-Giemsa stain, original magnification, x500).

osteosarcomas can be stained for alkaline phosphatase activity to increase the sensitivity and specificity of diagnosis. In dogs, alkaline phosphatase (ALP) staining resulted in 100% sensitivity and 89% specificity in differentiating osteosarcoma from other sarcomas.[21] It is critical to evaluate the sample cytologically first and diagnose a sarcoma before staining for ALP activity because reactive bone can stain positive for ALP just as easily as osteosarcoma.[4] Slides are incubated with nitroblue tetrazolium chloride/ 5-bromo-4-chloro-3-indolyl phosphate toluidine salt (NBT/BCIP) for 8 to 10 minutes. This material acts as the substrate for the ALP enzyme on the cell membrane. The initial studies with this substrate were performed on previously unstained slides; although a recent study found that previously stained slides can be destained and then incubated with NBT/BCIP.[22] Currently, cases of feline osteosarcoma are also being evaluated, and 7 feline osteosarcoma cases have been reviewed. All have been positive for ALP activity (Barger, unpublished data).

Synovial cell sarcomas share many of the features of other bone sarcomas (**Fig. 13**) and often are confused with histiocytic sarcomas, even with histopathology.[23]

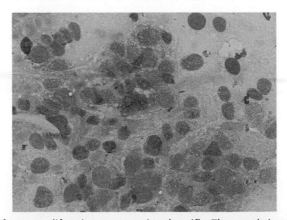

Fig. 13. Aspirate from a proliferative mass crossing the stifle. The sample is cellular and consists of a population of round to spindle-shaped cells. Diagnosis on cytology was a sarcoma, synovial cell sarcoma as the top differential because of the radiographic appearance. This diagnosis was confirmed with histopathology (Wright-Giemsa stain, original magnification, x500).

Distinguishing features include the radiographic appearance, because synovial cell sarcomas are known to cross the joint, and these tumors can have a biphasic appearance resulting in both mesenchymal and epithelial cells.[24] This feature can be identified cytologically as well.

Histiocytic sarcoma, including articular histiocytic sarcoma and hemophagocytic histiocytic sarcoma, can be diagnosed in bone. Breeds known to be predisposed to this tumor include Bernese mountain dogs, Rottweilers, golden retrievers, and flat-coated retrievers.[25] Cytologically, these tumors are highly cellular and exhibit marked cellular atypia. Erythrophagia is a common finding in hemophagocytic histiocytic sarcoma. These dogs are often profoundly anemic and can also have hypocholesterolemia.[25] These tumors can be distinguished from osteosarcoma with ALP staining because histiocytic sarcoma is negative for ALP activity.[21]

Hemangiosarcoma of bone has been reported, although bone is not considered a common location for this tumor.[26] Cytologically, these tumors are generally not very cellular. They arise from vascular endothelium and histopathologically are found to form vascular channels. Grossly, the tumors can be cavitated; therefore, it is difficult to find a solid and cellular area to aspirate. The cells are usually spindle shaped and plump. Epithelioid variants of the tumor have been reported.[27] Similar to histiocytic sarcoma, hemangiosarcoma is also negative for ALP activity. This finding can be useful in differentiating hemangiosarcoma from telangiectatic osteosarcoma.

Tumors of bone marrow origin include lymphoma and plasma cell neoplasia. Plasma cell tumors involving bone are usually a malignant variant of this tumor, multiple myeloma. Identification of punched out lesions in the bone, radiographically, are one of the criteria of diagnosis of this neoplasm.[28] Cytologically, aspirates of these bone lesions are highly cellular and consist of a population of neoplastic round cells. These cells have a moderate rim of basophilic cytoplasm and eccentrically placed nuclei. Often, a perinuclear clearing is observed consistent with a prominent Golgi apparatus (**Fig. 14**). In cats, cytology of multiple myeloma has revealed atypical plasma cells including multiple nuclei, clefted nuclei, anisocytosis and anisokaryosis.[29] Cells have also been described to have brightly eosinophilic cytoplasm.

Lymphoma of bone is fairly uncommon but has been reported.[30,31] Cytologically, lymphoma of the bone appears similar to lymphoma in other locations. A uniform population of neoplastic lymphocytes is observed. These cells have a scant rim of

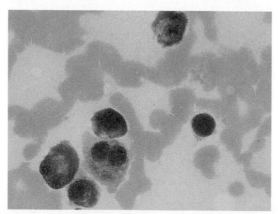

Fig. 14. Aspirate from a rib mass in a dog. The sample consisted of a pure population of neoplastic plasma cells. Binucleated cells were noted (Wright-Giemsa stain, original magnification, x1000).

cytoplasm with large round nuclei that fill the cytoplasm. The size of the cells can vary, as does the presence of prominent nucleoli. Immunophenotyping of the tumors is beneficial to determine T- or B-cell origin.

Tumors that metastasize to bone include squamous cell carcinoma (SCC), prostatic adenocarcinoma, transitional cell carcinoma, mammary gland adenocarcinoma, and thyroid carcinoma. Mechanisms for tumors to metastasize to bone include local invasion and hematogenous spread with migration into the marrow. SCC is known to invade bone. SCC is one of the most common oral tumors of cats.[32] SCCs arise from soft tissue but can invade local bone, so they often cause significant disease in the maxilla and mandible. Neoplastic squamous epithelial cells are known to express multiple factors that can increase osteoclast activity and proliferation such as receptor activator of nuclear factor kappa-B ligand,[33,34] parathyroid hormone-related protein, interleukin-6 and tumor necrosis factor-α.[35] Cytologically, aspirates are cellular and consist of clusters of neoplastic epithelial cells. These cells are often quite large, and many cells exhibit features similar to differentiated squamous epithelial cells, including keratinized cytoplasm and centrally placed nuclei. These cells also exhibit marked criteria of malignancy including large nuclei with prominent nucleoli, anisocytosis, and anisokaryosis. Perinuclear vacuolization is another common finding in these tumors (**Fig. 15**).

Other tumors metastasize to bone via the hematogenous route. The bone marrow is considered an appropriate environment for the neoplastic cells to proliferate.[35] These tumors can elicit an osteolytic or osteoproliferative response, which can result in significant pain and potentially pathologic fracture. Cytologic diagnosis can be made by aspirating the lytic lesion or aspirating marrow from an affected bone, although the former will likely be more effective. Clusters of neoplastic epithelial cells are observed, exhibiting marked criteria of malignancy (**Fig. 16**). Without knowledge of the source of the primary tumor, it is challenging to differentiate these tumors beyond metastatic carcinoma because the cells are often poorly differentiated. Often, a combination of clusters and loosely arranged cells can be identified. The presence of glandular structures, like acinar structures or markedly vacuolated cytoplasm of cells in clusters, makes diagnosis of metastatic carcinoma easier. Use of cytology for aspiration of a single lesion in an otherwise quiescent tumor may be the first indication of recurrence or metastases.[36]

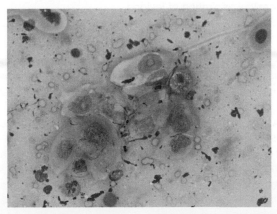

Fig. 15. Aspirate from a mandibular mass in a cat. Clusters of neoplastic squamous cells are pictured. These cells are large with a centrally placed round nucleus and prominent nucleoli (Wright-Giemsa stain, original magnification, x500).

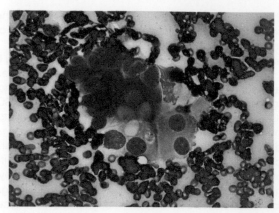

Fig. 16. Aspiration of a small lytic lesion in the lumbar vertebrate from a neutered male golden retriever. Pictured is a cluster of neoplastic epithelial cells occasionally containing eosinophilic product within the cytoplasm. This sample is suggestive of metastatic prostatic or transitional cell carcinoma. On rectal palpation, a large prostatic mass was palpated and aspirated with a diagnosis of carcinoma (Wright-Giemsa stain, original magnification, x500).

BENIGN LYTIC LESIONS

Aneurysmal bone cysts are benign but locally destructive lesions. Histologically, these lesions consist of fibrous connective tissue with many multinucleated giant cells and few inflammatory cells. Cytologically, these structures can be surprisingly cellular and consist of multinucleated giant cells, scattered histiocytic cells, and aggregates of spindle shaped cells.[37] Radiographic evaluation is critical to accurately diagnose an aneurysmal bone cyst.

SUMMARY

Aspiration of bone lesions can be very rewarding and is beneficial in differentiating inflammatory from neoplastic processes. Cytology is a component of the diagnostic process and should be combined with signalment, history, and radiographic findings to come to a final diagnosis. Different techniques and imaging modalities are available to assist with successful aspiration of lesions.

REFERENCES

1. Domanski HA, Akerman M, Carlen B, et al. Core-needle biopsy performed by the cytopathologist. Cancer 2005;105(4):229–39.
2. Agarwal S, Agarwal T, Agarwal R, et al. Fine needle aspiration of bone tumors. Cancer Detect Prev 2000;24(6):602–9.
3. Domanski HA, Akerman M. Fine-needle aspiration of primary osteosarcoma: a cytological-histological study. Diagn Cytopathol 2005;32(5):269–75.
4. Britt T, Clifford C, Barger A. Diagnosing appendicular osteosarcoma with ultrasound-guided fine-needle aspiration: 36 cases. J Small Anim Pract 2007;48(3):145–50.
5. Cohen M, Bohling MC, Wright JC, et al. Evaluation of sensitivity and specificity of cytologic examination: 269 cases (1999-2000). J Am Vet Med Assoc 2003;222(7): 964–7.
6. Handa U, Bal A, Mohan H, et al. Fine needle aspiration cytology in the diagnosis of bone lesions. Cytopathology 2005;16:59–64.

7. Hostettler FC, Wiener DJ, Welle MM, et al. Post mortem computed tomography and core needle biopsy in comparison to autopsy in eleven Bernese mountain dogs with histiocytic sarcoma. BMC Vet Res 2015;11:229–39.

8. Neihaus SA, Locke JE, Barger AM. A novel method of core aspirate cytology compared to fine-needle aspiration of diagnosing osteosarcoma. J Am Anim Hosp Assoc 2011;47(5):317–23.

9. Weisbrode SE. Bone and joints. In: McGavin MD, Zachary JF, editors. Pathologic basis of veterinary disease. 4th edition. St Louis (MO): Mosby Elsevier; 2007. p. 1041–106.

10. Akerman M, Domanski HA, Jonsson K. Cytology of normal constituents in bone aspirates and of reactive changes. Monogr Clin Cytol 2010;19:13–7.

11. Salas EN, Royal D, Kurz L, et al. Osteomyelitis associated with *Nocardiopsis composta* in a dog. Can Vet J 2015;56(5):466–70.

12. Hilligas J, Van Wie E, Bar J, et al. Vertebral osteomyelitis and multiple cutaneous lesions in a dog caused by Nocardia pseudobrasiliensis. J Vet Intern Med 2014; 28:1621–5.

13. Erne JB, Walker MC, Strik N, et al. Systemic infection with Geomyces organisms in a dog with lytic bone lesions. J Am Vet Med Assoc 2007;230(4):537–40.

14. Oshin A, Griffon D, Lemberger K, et al. Patellar blastomycosis in a dog. J Am Anim Hosp Assoc 2009;45(5):239–44.

15. Headley SA, Mota FC, Lindsay S, et al. *Cryptococcus neoformans* var. *grubii*-induced arthritis with encephalitic dissemination in a dog and review of published literature. Mycopathologia 2016;181(7–8):595–601.

16. Shimokawa Miyama T, Umeki S, Baba K, et al. Neutropenia associated with osteomyelitis du to *Hepatozoon canis* infection in a dog. J Vet Med Sci 2011;73(10): 1389–93.

17. Lin TY, Hosoya K, Drost WT, et al. What is your diagnosis? Fine-needle aspirate of an aggressive bone lesion in a dog. Vet Clin Pathol 2010;39:397–8.

18. Waltman SS, Seguin B, Cooper BJ, et al. Clinical outcome of nonnasal chondrosarcoma in dogs: thirty one cases (1986-2003). Vet Surg 2007;36:266–71.

19. Reinhardt S, Stockhaus C, Teske E, et al. Assessment of cytological criteria for diagnosing osteosarcoma in dogs. J Small Anim Pract 2005;46(2):65–70.

20. Barger AM, Skowronski MC, MacNeill AL. Cytologic identification of erythrophagocytic neoplasms in dogs. Vet Clin Pathol 2012;41(4):587–9.

21. Barger A, Graca R, Bailey K, et al. Use of alkaline phosphatase staining to differentiate canine osteosarcoma from other vimentin-positive tumors. Vet Pathol 2005;42:161–5.

22. Ryseff JK, Bohn AA. Detection of alkaline phosphatase in canine cells previously stained with Wright-Giemsa and its utility in differentiating osteosarcoma from other mesenchymal tumors. Vet Clin Pathol 2012;41:391–5.

23. Craig LE, Julian ME, Ferracone JD. The diagnosis and prognosis of synovial tumors in dogs: 35 cases. Vet Pathol 2002;39:66–73.

24. Loukopoulos P, Heng HG, Arshad H. Canine biphasic synovial sarcoma: case report and immunohistochemical characterization. J Vet Sci 2004;5(2):173–80.

25. Moore PF. A review of histiocytic diseases of dogs and cats. Vet Pathol 2014; 51(1):167–84.

26. Smith AN. Hemangiosarcoma in dogs and cats. Vet Clin Small Anim 2003;33: 533–52.

27. Warren AL, Summers BA. Epithelioid variant of hemangioma and hemangiosarcoma in the dog, horse and cow. Vet Pathol 2007;44(1):15–24.

28. Sternberg R, Wypij J, Barger AM. An overview of multiple myeloma in dogs and cats. Vet Med 2009;104:468–76.

29. Patel RT, Caceres A, French AF, et al. Multiple myeloma in 16 cats: a retrospective study. Vet Clin Pathol 2005;34(4):341–52.

30. Brockley LK, Heading KL, Jardine JE, et al. Polyostotic lymphoma with multiple pathological fractures in a six-month-old cat. J Feline Med Surg 2012;14(4): 285–91.

31. Ito T, Hisasue M, Neo S, et al. A case of atypical canine lymphoma with oral mass and multiple osteolysis. J Vet Med Sci 2007;69(9):977–80.

32. Wypij JM, Fan TM, Fredrickson RL, et al. In vivo and in vitro efficacy of Zoledronate for treating oral squamous cell carcinoma in cats. J Vet Intern Med 2008;22: 158–63.

33. Barger AM, Fan TM, de Lorimier L-P, et al. Expression of receptor activator of nuclear factor κ-B ligand (RANKL) in neoplasms of dogs and cats. J Vet Intern Med 2007;21:133–40.

34. Jimi E, Shin M, Furuta H, et al. The RANKL/RANK system as a therapeutic target for bon invasion by oral squamous cell carcinoma. Int J Oncol 2013;42(3):803–9.

35. Simmons JK, Hildreth BE, Supsavhad W, et al. Animal models of bone metastasis. Vet Pathol 2015;52(5):827–41.

36. Akerman M, Domanski HA, Jonsson K. Bone metastases. Monogr Clin Cytol 2010;19:75–80.

37. Akerman M, Domanski HA, Jonsson K. Cytological features of bone tumors in FNA smears V: giant-cell lesions. Monogr Clin Cytol 2010;19:55–61.

Cytology of Skin Neoplasms

Mark C. Johnson, DVM*, Alexandra N. Myers, DVM

KEYWORDS

- Fine-needle aspiration • Skin mass • Cytology • Cutaneous • Neoplasm

KEY POINTS

- Cytology is a useful, first-line diagnostic tool for differentiating skin neoplasms and may allow for rapid diagnosis and initiation of treatment.
- Clinical history, signalment, and precise localization of the mass should be considered when evaluating cytology of skin masses.
- Skin neoplasms can typically be classified as benign or malignant and divided into one of 3 categories: epithelial, mesenchymal, and round cell.
- Cytology has its limitations, and veterinarians and owners should be aware that biopsy and histologic evaluation may be needed for definitive diagnosis and malignancy evaluation.

INTRODUCTION

Fine-needle aspiration (FNA) with cytologic evaluation of skin masses is an important diagnostic option for veterinarians, as it has the potential to provide vital information for treatment considerations. Cytologic evaluation may allow the veterinarian to rule out inflammatory causes for the mass and identify the general category and often the specific type of tumor that is present.

Veterinarians should be aware that there are limitations to interpreting cytology samples. Cells obtained by FNA may not be representative of all cells in the mass. Likewise, cytology should be used cautiously to determine the malignancy potential of skin tumors, as not all malignant tumors display notable cellular atypia and not all benign tumors display minimal cellular atypia. Additionally, inflammation can induce epithelial and mesenchymal cells to undergo hyperplasia or dysplasia, which can mimic neoplastic transformation in cytology samples.

Neoplasms of the skin are cytologically divided into epithelial, mesenchymal, and round cell tumors, based on their cell of origin. Cytologic features for each of these

The authors have nothing to disclose.
Department of Veterinary Pathobiology, College of Veterinary Medicine and Biomedical Sciences, Texas A&M University, Mail Stop 4467, College Station, TX 77843-4467, USA
* Corresponding author.
E-mail address: mjohnson@cvm.tamu.edu

Vet Clin Small Anim 47 (2017) 85–110
http://dx.doi.org/10.1016/j.cvsm.2016.07.006
0195-5616/17/© 2016 Elsevier Inc. All rights reserved.
vetsmall.theclinics.com

categories are provided to aid in the classification process and the identification of specific tumors. The intent of these sections is to familiarize veterinarians with the more common tumors of the skin.

CUTANEOUS EPITHELIAL TUMORS

Epithelial cells tend to exfoliate well with FNA and have a clustering appearance.[1] There are exceptions, as keratinized squamous epithelial cells (keratinocytes) can cluster or be solitary in nature (**Fig. 1**).[1] The amount of cytoplasm can vary from scant in basilar cells to abundant in keratinocytes. Epithelial cells are often round to oval but can be polygonal or columnar.[1]

Follicular Cysts

Follicular cysts originate from the epithelium of the hair follicle and include infundibular follicular cysts (epidermal inclusion cysts), isthmus catagen cysts, hair bulb matrical cysts, and pan-follicular cysts.[2] These cysts are frequently seen in dogs, with predisposed breeds including the boxer, Doberman pinscher, miniature schnauzer and shih tzu.[2] Follicular cysts are also reported in cats.[3] Grossly, cysts will often appear as a small, cutaneous, often hairless mass that can have a central pore filled with pale white to grey-black, waxy, keratinaceous material.[2] Manual expression of this material should be discouraged, as cysts can rupture with pressure. The cyst material can induce severe localized inflammation when released into the dermis and subcutaneous tissue.[2]

Cytologic examination of cysts often reveals large amounts of amorphous keratin debris with occasional cholesterol crystals (**Fig. 2**).[4] As these cysts are lined by epithelium, few basilar-type epithelial cells can be observed in these samples; however, if large numbers of basilar cells are noted, more consideration should be given to a hair follicle tumor (**Fig. 3**). Neutrophils, macrophages, and multinucleated giant cells may be seen if inflammation is present (**Fig. 4**).

Hair Follicle Tumors

Hair follicle tumors originate from the different regions of the follicular epithelium and include tricholemmoma, trichofolliculoma, trichoepithelioma, and pilomatricoma.[2]

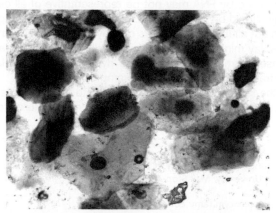

Fig. 1. Skin mass. FNA. Dog. Numerous, solitary keratinocytes are round to polygonal in shape with medium blue cytoplasm and a small condensed nucleus (Diff-Quik, original magnification ×60).

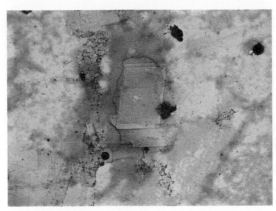

Fig. 2. Follicular cyst. FNA. Dog. Several, large, clear cholesterol crystals are present. Cholesterol crystals in skin masses are not pathognomonic for follicular cysts or hair follicle tumors, but their presence should increase the index of suspicion for these tumors (Diff-Quik, original magnification ×60).

Infundibular keratinizing acanthoma is an additional tumor considered to originate from the hair follicle in dogs. Hair follicle tumors are common in many breeds of dogs but are less frequent in cats. Like cysts, hair follicle tumors are typically solitary, alopecic skin masses that have a superficial epidermal component, often with keratin debris present within the center of the mass. These tumors are usually benign; but malignant forms rarely occur, most commonly with pilomatricoma.[5–8]

Differentiating the various follicular tumors from each other and from cysts is challenging with cytologic evaluation, and biopsy with histologic evaluation is usually required for definitive diagnosis. Cytologic features observed in hair follicle tumors include keratinocytes, keratin debris, numerous basilar type epithelial cells, and ghost epithelial cells (see **Fig. 1**; **Figs. 5** and **6**).[9,10] Ghost cells are follicular basilar cells with a transparent or fading nucleus that are typically only observed in trichoepitheliomas, pilomatricomas, and matrical cysts.[2] Few sebaceous epithelial cells can be observed;

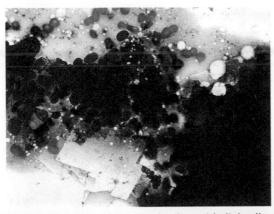

Fig. 3. Hair follicle tumor. FNA. Dog. Numerous basilar epithelial cells with round to oval nuclei and scant amounts of light blue cytoplasm are admixed with several, clear cholesterol crystals and occasional erythrocytes (Diff-Quik, original magnification ×60).

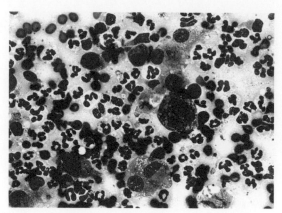

Fig. 4. Ruptured follicular cyst. FNA. Dog. Pyogranulomatous inflammation secondary to rupture of a follicular cyst. Note the large numbers of neutrophils, macrophages, and rare multinucleated giant cells (Diff-Quik, original magnification ×60).

but if large numbers of these are present, a sebaceous gland tumor should be considered.

Cutaneous Basilar Epithelial Tumors

These neoplasms are composed of small basilar epithelial cells without associated keratinization. Most of these tumors in dogs are now classified as trichoblastomas when biopsy with histologic evaluation is performed. Basal cell tumors in cats are also included in this category. Although these neoplasms have similar morphologic features, basal cell tumors are thought to originate from the pluripotent basal cells of the epidermis, whereas trichoblastomas are thought to originate from the germ cells of the hair follicle.[2,9,11–13]

Basal cell tumors are relatively common in cats with Persian, Himalayan, and Siamese breeds predisposed.[2] Trichoblastomas are seen in cats and dogs, most notably in poodles and cocker spaniels.[2] Both of these neoplasms are often solitary, raised,

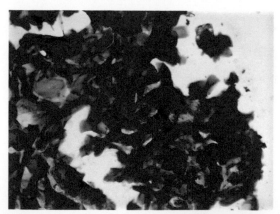

Fig. 5. Hair follicle tumor. FNA. Dog. Large amounts of keratin debris are present, which is a cytologic feature of both hair follicle tumors and follicular cysts (Diff-Quik, original magnification ×60).

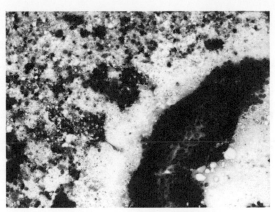

Fig. 6. Hair follicle tumor. FNA. Dog. A large sheet of basilar epithelial cells is present along with keratin debris (Diff-Quik, original magnification ×20).

nonhaired skin masses that are commonly located on the ears, neck, and forelimbs. In cats, they may be ulcerated, hairless, or pedunculated with dark blue to black pigmentation.[2,9] Cutaneous basilar epithelial neoplasms are predominantly benign tumors, but malignancies do occur, such as basal cell carcinoma.

Cytologically, these tumors are composed of numerous clusters of basilar-type epithelial cells, which are characterized by small size and a high nuclear to cytoplasmic ratio (**Fig. 7**). Because these tumors do not undergo follicular or epithelial keratinization, numerous keratinocytes, keratin debris, and ghost epithelial cells should not be observed. Similar to hair follicle tumors, histologic evaluation is needed to differentiate these neoplasms. Basal cell carcinoma is associated with increased cytologic criteria of malignancy in neoplastic cells (**Fig. 8**).

Sebaceous Gland Tumors

Tumors of the sebaceous glands are common in dogs but infrequent in cats, with Persians having a higher predisposition.[2,9] Sebaceous gland tumors are subdivided into nodular sebaceous hyperplasia, sebaceous gland adenoma, sebaceous gland

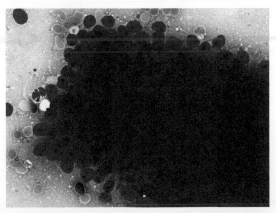

Fig. 7. Cutaneous basilar epithelial tumor. FNA. Dog. Note the numerous basilar epithelial cells from a presumptive trichoblastoma (Diff-Quik, original magnification x60).

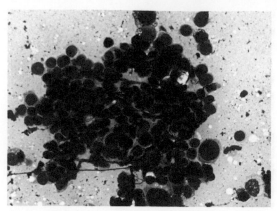

Fig. 8. Basal cell carcinoma. FNA. Cat. A cluster of basilar epithelial cells with notable anisokaryosis within several cells on the edge of the clusters (Diff-Quik, original magnification ×60).

epithelioma, and sebaceous gland adenocarcinoma. Nodular sebaceous hyperplasia is the most common sebaceous tumor in dogs, noted frequently in cocker spaniels, beagles, dachshunds, poodles, and miniature schnauzers.[2] Sebaceous adenoma and nodular sebaceous hyperplasia are common on the head, eyelids, limbs, and trunk. A sebaceous adenoma that is associated with the meibomian glands of the eyelid is referred to as a *meibomian gland adenoma*. Sebaceous neoplasms are small, irregular, protruding, or wartlike, variably pigmented skin masses that are sometimes covered with a waxy, crusty exudate. Sebaceous gland epithelioma is a less common variant of sebaceous gland tumors and is often located on the eyelids and head.[2] Sebaceous gland adenocarcinomas are rare but, when present, are often ulcerated and larger than their benign counterparts.

Cytology samples from nodular sebaceous hyperplasia and sebaceous adenoma have clusters of epithelial cells containing abundant, foamy cytoplasm and small, condensed nuclei (**Fig. 9**). Sebaceous epithelioma differs in that numerous basilar epithelial cells with occasional foamy-appearing sebaceous cells are noted in cytology preparations. Sebaceous gland adenocarcinoma will often have similar foamy cells, but notable cytologic atypia is expected in the epithelial cells (**Fig. 10**). Like other

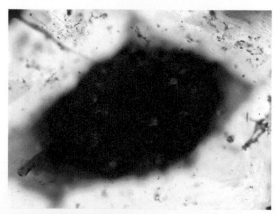

Fig. 9. Sebaceous gland adenoma. FNA. Dog. Sebaceous epithelial cells with foamy cytoplasm and a small, condensed nucleus (Diff-Quik, original magnification ×60).

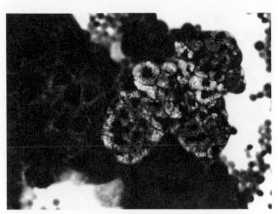

Fig. 10. Sebaceous gland adenocarcinoma. FNA. Dog. A large sheet of epithelial cells displaying notable cytologic criteria of malignancy to include binucleation and multinucleation, anisokaryosis, and increased nuclear to cytoplasmic ratios. Note the small cluster of more normal-appearing sebaceous epithelial cells in the center of the image (Diff-Quik, original magnification ×60).

epithelial tumors, histologic evaluation is often needed to differentiate the types of sebaceous gland neoplasms.

Perianal Gland Tumors

Perianal gland tumors are typically benign and are considered modified sebaceous gland neoplasms. They are most commonly noted in intact, older male dogs and are known to express both androgen and estrogen receptors, but they can also occur in adult neutered male dogs and adult spayed and intact female dogs.[14] Cocker spaniels, English bulldogs, Samoyeds, Siberian huskies, Afghans, dachshunds, German shepherds, shih tzus and Lhaso apsos are predisposed to these tumors.[2] These tumors are not seen in cats. Perianal gland adenomas can vary grossly from a small, solitary, raised skin mass on the perineum to a swollen, circumferential, ulcerated mass involving the entire perineum. Additionally, these neoplasms can be located in the skin on the tail, prepuce, upper rear limbs, and dorsal lumbosacral regions.[2] It can be challenging to differentiate perianal gland hyperplasia from perianal gland adenomas based on gross appearance. Perianal gland carcinomas are rarely reported.[15]

Cytologically, these tumors are composed of numerous hepatoid epithelial cells arranged in dense clusters. These cells are named for their often-striking resemblance to hepatocytes. This appearance is characterized by abundant, medium blue, granular cytoplasm with a centrally located nucleus and a single prominent nucleolus. In most cases, variable numbers of basilar epithelial cells, often referred to as *reserve cells*, are arranged around the periphery of the clusters of hepatoid cells (**Figs. 11** and **12**).[9,16] When only reserve cells are noted cytologically, this tumor can be mistaken for the apocrine gland adenocarcinoma of the anal sac (anal sac adenocarcinoma).

Apocrine Gland Tumors

These tumors are divided into anal sac adenocarcinoma, ceruminous gland adenoma and adenocarcinoma of the ear canal, and sweat gland tumors.

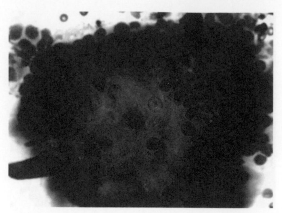

Fig. 11. Perianal gland tumor. FNA. Dog. A large group of hepatoid epithelial cells is in the left center of the image. Note the small reserve cells at the upper right corner of the image with small round nuclei and minimal cytoplasm (Diff-Quik, original magnification ×60).

Anal sac adenocarcinoma

Anal sac adenocarcinoma is seen primarily in dogs and can be associated with paraneoplastic hypercalcemia due to the high levels of circulating parathyroid-related peptide in these dogs.[17–19]

Cytologically, anal sac adenocarcinoma is most often composed of numerous round to oval, bare nuclei (**Fig. 13**). When these cells are found intact, they are basilar in appearance, with scant amounts of pale blue to clear cytoplasm and a small round to oval nucleus. These cells generally exhibit minimal cytologic atypia despite their malignant biological behavior.

Ceruminous gland tumors

Ceruminous gland adenomas and adenocarcinomas are more commonly reported in cats but can be seen in dogs.[20,21] These tumors originate from specialized apocrine

Fig. 12. Perianal gland tumor. FNA. Dog. Large cluster of perianal gland epithelial cells with few hepatoid epithelial cells and a predominance of small reserve epithelial cells (Diff-Quik, original magnification ×20).

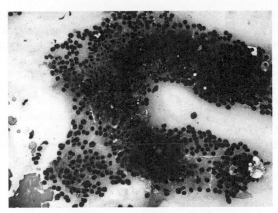

Fig. 13. Anal sac adenocarcinoma. FNA. Dog. A large aggregate of neoplastic epithelial cells with a predominance of bare, round nuclei in a proteinaceous background. Note that the nuclei do not display significant atypia, despite the malignant nature of this tumor. The light pink material is likely collagen from supporting stroma within the tumor (Diff-Quik, original magnification ×20).

sweat glands within the ear canal and often appear clinically as a pedunculated or lobulated mass within the ear canal.

Cytologically, large amounts of amorphous to granular, blue-grey debris may be present in addition to variable numbers of epithelial cells. Epithelial cells can be arranged in linear arrays or clusters and are variably round to columnar with a moderate amount of light blue cytoplasm that occasionally contains dark blue to black granular pigment, which can be mistaken for melanin (**Fig. 14**).[9,21] More notable cellular atypia is observed with ceruminous gland adenocarcinoma, but histologic evaluation is usually needed to determine the malignancy potential.

Sweat gland tumors
Sweat gland tumors are less common than sebaceous or basal cell neoplasms in dogs and cats and may be located adjacent to the paw pads or on the head, neck, back,

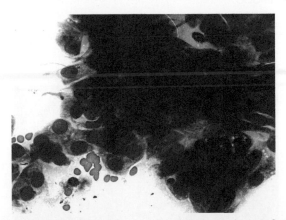

Fig. 14. Ceruminous gland adenocarcinoma. FNA. Cat. A dense cluster of round to columnar neoplastic epithelial cells is present in haphazard and linear arrays. Note that many of the cells contain numerous, dark blue to black, intracytoplasmic granules. This pigment can be confused with melanin (Diff-Quik, original magnification ×60).

and flanks.[22,23] These tumors are typically benign and are composed of several subtypes that cannot be distinguished cytologically (apocrine cysts, apocrine cystadenomas, apocrine secretory adenomas, and apocrine ductular adenomas).[22] Malignant tumors of the sweat glands and their ducts are uncommon.[23] The gross appearance of both benign and malignant forms may vary widely. They may be cystic to nodular, firm to fluctuant, and variably sized. Cystic varieties may have a blue or purple hue when observed grossly.[22]

Cytologically, these tumors are composed of round to cuboidal epithelial cells that can be arranged in linear arrays or in small clusters. In benign tumors, these cells have small to moderate amounts of medium blue, smooth to finely granular cytoplasm with an eccentrically placed, round nucleus and a small, round nucleolus. Malignant sweat gland tumors are expected to exhibit significant cytologic criteria of malignancy.

Papilloma

Squamous papilloma is a common cutaneous neoplasm in dogs, with 5 different variants noted.[2] It is more common in male dogs, and cocker spaniels and Kerry blue terriers have a higher predilection for this neoplasm.[2] Papillomas are also reported in cats.[24,25] Papillomavirus is a known cause for papillomas in dogs and cats, but it is unclear if the virus is responsible for all cases.[24–29]

Papillomas can be solitary or multiple, cutaneous or mucocutaneous masses with a crusty, wartlike appearance, which correlates with the epithelial hyperplasia and hyperkeratosis observed on hematoxylin and eosin (H&E)–stained sections (**Fig. 15**). Intranuclear viral inclusions can occasionally be observed in squamous epithelial cells on H&E histologic sections (**Fig. 16**). Histologic evaluation is usually needed for a definitive diagnosis of papilloma and to exclude squamous cell carcinoma (SCC) as a possibility. Papillomas can undergo malignant transformation to SCC.

Cytologic evaluation of these masses can reveal large numbers of nucleated keratinocytes that display some nuclear atypia, such as retention of a large nucleus and increased nuclear to cytoplasmic ratio (**Fig. 17**). Intranuclear viral inclusions are rarely observed in keratinocytes in cytology samples of papillomas. Papilloma will share similar cytologic features with SCC, although the atypia is expected to be more pronounced in SCC.

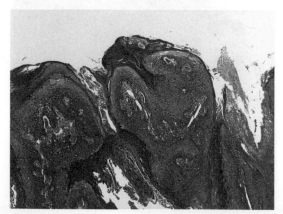

Fig. 15. Papilloma. Biopsy of digital mass. Dog. Note the wartlike appearance of a papilloma with epithelial hyperplasia and hyperkeratosis (hematoxylin-eosin, original magnification ×4).

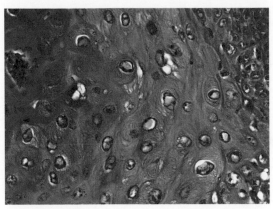

Fig. 16. Papilloma. Biopsy of digital mass. Dog. In the center of the image are 3, lightly amphophilic, smooth, intranuclear, papillomavirus inclusions that have displaced the chromatin to the periphery of the nucleus (hematoxylin-eosin, original magnification ×60).

Squamous Cell Carcinoma

SCC is a common malignant skin tumor in dogs and cats that is often induced by solar radiation exposure. Other risk factors for SCC are lack of skin pigmentation, sparse hair coat, and cutaneous papillomavirus infection.[2,30] It is more commonly seen in older animals, and white-haired cats have a significantly higher risk of developing SCC than other cats, most notably on the face.[2] Tumors may be solitary or multiple and can be located in various sites, including the face and ears, body, limbs, and digits. Grossly, masses can be proliferative, ulcerative, or both.

Cytologically, SCC is often composed of numerous keratinocytes that may or may not exhibit a cohesive nature (**Fig. 18**). Keratinocytes can display notable malignant features to include retention of large nuclei, nuclear fragmentation, binucleation or multinucleation, anisokaryosis, and nuclear to cytoplasmic asynchrony (see **Fig. 18**). Atypical parabasal or basal epithelial cells can also be observed as well as variable numbers of neutrophils (**Fig. 19**).

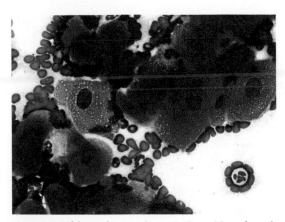

Fig. 17. Papilloma. Scraping of hyperkeratotic crust. Dog. Many keratinocytes with retention of large nuclei are present. Note the eosinophilic, finely vacuolated cytoplasm of many of these cells, likely secondary to cytoplasmic degeneration associated with a papillomavirus infection (Diff-Quik, original magnification ×60).

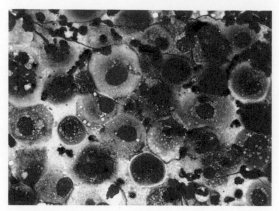

Fig. 18. SCC. FNA. Dog. Large numbers of atypical keratinocytes are present. Notable cytologic criteria of malignancy in these cells include retention of large nuclei, binucleation, and anisokaryosis (Diff-Quik, original magnification ×60).

CUTANEOUS MESENCHYMAL TUMORS

Mesenchymal tumors (also known as *spindle-cell tumors*) are a group of connective tissue tumors that may arise in the dermis or subcutaneous tissues. Cytologically, most types of mesenchymal cells have wispy or indistinct cytoplasmic borders and are spindled to stellate. The cells are most often arranged individually and do not form clusters as epithelial cells do. With FNA, masses composed of mesenchymal cells are often poorly cellular (ie, the cells do not exfoliate well); however, some mesenchymal tumors may be moderately to highly cellular, especially when poorly differentiated.

With cytologic evaluation alone, differentiating mesenchymal tumors from each other and from non-neoplastic lesions (eg, fibroplasia or granulation tissue) is difficult. This difficulty is partly because many of the mesenchymal tumors share similar morphologic features. Furthermore, even non-neoplastic mesenchymal cells, such

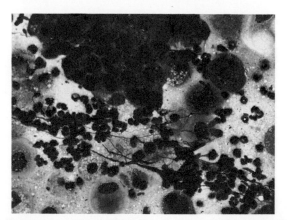

Fig. 19. SCC. FNA. Dog. A small cluster of parabasal epithelial cells is present at the top of the image. These cells and small, basal epithelial cells are often seen in cytologic samples from SCC, in addition to the keratinocytes. Note that numerous degenerate neutrophils and occasional atypical keratinocytes are also present (Diff-Quik, original magnification ×60).

as fibroblasts in a reactive lesion, can display marked atypia. A common pitfall of examining mesenchymal cells is to misclassify reactive lesions as malignant, which may lead to unnecessary and invasive treatments. Biopsy with histopathology is often required to accurately classify masses containing mesenchymal cells. That said, cytology can be helpful for rapidly diagnosing mesenchymal neoplasia when certain cytologic characteristics are observed, as described next.

Lipoma

Lipomas are benign neoplasms of fat (adipocytes). They are very common in dogs and uncommon in other species.[31] These neoplasms may be single or multiple, soft, subcutaneous masses occurring on the thorax, abdomen, and upper limbs.[9] When aspirated material is expelled onto a slide, the droplets appear greasy and will not dry.[9]

Cytologic evaluation of a lipoma may reveal scattered aggregates of adipocytes admixed with few spindle cells and bare nuclei (**Fig. 20**). Adipocytes may also be seen with aspiration of normal subcutaneous fat, as might be present around a lymph node or tumor. Rarely, a mass that is consistent with a lipoma on physical examination may actually represent or conceal a tumor of greater clinical significance (eg, mast cell tumor [MCT]), so aspiration of these masses is always recommended. If necessary, surgical excision may be performed and is usually curative, though infiltrative lipomas may be difficult to resect and may recur.[9]

Quick tip

The methanol fixative (step 1) of rapid cytologic stains (eg, Diff-Quik) and other Romanowsky-type stains can dissolve lipid, yielding an acellular slide.[9] If a lipoma is suspected based on the greasy, nondrying nature of the aspirate, the methanol fixative may be skipped and the slide dipped gently in the red and purple stains as usual. This technique may help to preserve any adipocytes on the slide.

Soft Tissue Sarcoma

Soft tissue sarcomas are a group of mesenchymal neoplasms that appear morphologically similar when evaluated cytologically.[32] In addition, the tumors in this category are similar in terms of clinical progression, metastasis, and treatment considerations. For these reasons, a specific diagnosis of tumor type beyond that of soft tissue

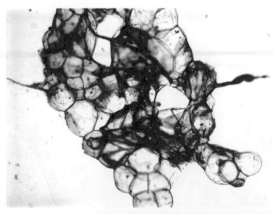

Fig. 20. Lipoma. FNA. Dog. Large, clear cells (adipocytes) with small nuclei are typically found in aggregates such as this one. Aspirates of a lipoma may also be acellular (Diff-Quik, original magnification ×20).

sarcoma is not clinically necessary.[32] As a group, these neoplasms are generally considered to be locally invasive with a low to moderate metastatic potential.[32] Although many mesenchymal neoplasms are derived from soft tissues, only the following neoplasms are routinely termed *soft tissue sarcomas* in the literature.[32,33]

- Fibrosarcoma
- Myxosarcoma
- Peripheral nerve sheath tumors (excluding brachial plexus tumors)
- Perivascular wall tumors
- Liposarcoma

It is not always possible to distinguish between soft tissue sarcomas, other mesenchymal neoplasms, and non-neoplastic proliferations of mesenchymal cells (eg, granulation tissue); therefore, the terms *mesenchymal proliferation* or *mesenchymal neoplasm* may be the most specific cytologic interpretation possible. Biopsy with histologic examination is often required to distinguish between these processes and to rule out a sarcoma with more aggressive biologic behavior (eg, hemangiosarcoma).[33]

The cytologic characteristics of the individual types of soft tissue sarcomas are discussed next. These characteristics may allow differentiation of a soft tissue sarcoma from mesenchymal proliferation or more aggressive sarcoma.

Fibrosarcoma

Fibrosarcomas are uncommon in dogs but relatively more common in cats.[34] They may arise at any anatomic site with a predilection for trunk and legs.[34] Vaccine-associated fibrosarcomas in cats are locally invasive and aggressive neoplasms.[34] In general, fibrosarcomas are typically firm and poorly circumscribed and may be multilobular, alopecic, and/or ulcerated.[34] Cytologically, fibrosarcomas consist of plump, spindled cells arranged individually or in aggregates associated with extracellular, pink, collagenous material (**Fig. 21**).[9] Nuclei are typically elongated and display marked pleomorphism.[9]

Myxosarcoma

Myxomas and myxosarcomas are rare tumors in dogs and cats.[34] They usually present as a single, soft, infiltrative, poorly circumscribed mass on the limbs, thorax, or

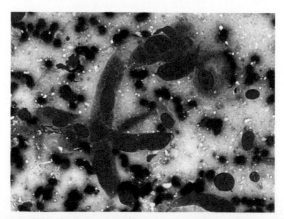

Fig. 21. Fibrosarcoma. FNA. Dog. Large, elongated neoplastic fibroblasts display multiple characteristics of malignancy, including multi-nucleation, multiple and variably sized nucleoli, and anisokaryosis (Diff-Quik, original magnification ×60).

abdomen. Myxosarcomas are distinguished cytologically from other mesenchymal neoplasms by the presence of abundant, pink, extracellular, amorphous, and mucinous matrix material.[9] Cells are spindled to stellate and often exhibit *windrowing*, an appearance created when cells line up in rows because of the high viscosity of the mucinous material.[35]

Liposarcoma
Liposarcomas are rare, malignant neoplasms of adipocytes. Their gross appearance is variable: some may resemble lipomas, whereas others may be firm, poorly circum-scribed, grey-white, subcutaneous masses that infiltrate adjacent tissues.[31] They may occur anywhere on the body and have a moderate metastatic potential.[9] Several sub-types of liposarcoma exist that have varying histologic appearances[31]; thus, the cyto-logic appearance can be expected to vary as well. Liposarcomas may be highly cellular and composed of plump, spindled cells with distinct, clear lipid vacuoles in the cytoplasm.[9] Other liposarcomas have a more round-cell appearance with abun-dant cytoplasm containing few or no vacuoles (**Fig. 22**A). Typically, a large number of lipid vacuoles (free lipid) are present in the background.

Care should be taken to differentiate inflamed or necrotic fat from a liposarcoma. The distinction can be difficult to make, as lipid vacuoles are a prominent feature in both conditions. Additionally, macrophages, multinucleated giant cells, and immature adipocytes can mimic neoplastic cells (see **Fig. 22**B). Biopsy with histologic evaluation is typically recommended when the distinction is unclear.

Perivascular wall tumors and peripheral nerve sheath tumors
Perivascular wall tumors (including hemangiopericytoma) and peripheral nerve sheath tumors (excluding those of the brachial plexus and spinal nerve roots) often have a similar cytologic appearance. Grossly, they are often firm, multilobular, subcutaneous to dermal masses that are most commonly found on the limbs or trunk. Generally, these tumors are locally aggressive but have modest metastatic potential.[32] Perivas-cular wall tumors and peripheral nerve sheath tumors may consist predominantly of

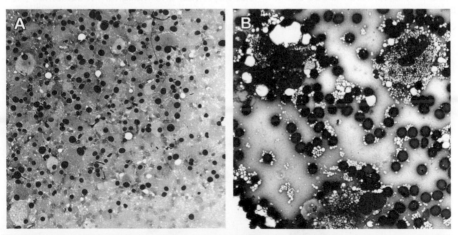

Fig. 22. Comparison of liposarcoma and reactive fat (panniculitis). (*A*) Liposarcoma. FNA. Dog. This liposarcoma is composed of large, rounded cells with abundant cytoplasm and few cytoplasmic vacuoles. Abundant, clear vacuoles in the background represent free lipid (Wright stain, original magnification ×20). (*B*) Panniculitis. Foamy, multinucleated macro-phages may be mistaken for neoplastic cells (Diff-Quik, original magnification ×60).

stellate cells with round to oval nuclei and moderate amounts of pale, wispy, veil-like cytoplasm. Crown cells (multinucleated neoplastic cells with a ring of nuclei) are a unique feature observed occasionally with these tumors (**Fig. 23**).[9,36]

Hemangiosarcoma/Hemangioma

Hemangiosarcoma is a malignant neoplasm of endothelial cells that line blood vessels, and hemangioma is its benign counterpart. These neoplasms are common in dogs and less common in cats.[31] Cutaneous hemangiosarcoma may represent metastasis from a primary visceral tumor; alternatively, it may be a primary neoplasm with origins in the dermis or subcutis. Primary *dermal* hemangiosarcoma and hemangioma have been associated with exposure to solar radiation and are seen most commonly in the lightly pigmented skin of the abdomen and prepuce.[37] These masses typically present as small, raised, dark red to purple nodules. *Subcutaneous* hemangiosarcoma, on the other hand, has no site predilection and often behaves more aggressively.[37] These hemangiosarcomas commonly present as larger, soft to fluctuant masses with a bruiselike appearance.[38]

Cytologically, hemangiosarcoma has a variable appearance and may be indistinguishable from other sarcomas.[39] Cellularity ranges from low to high, and hemodilution is a consistent feature. Cells are typically pleomorphic and exhibit marked anisocytosis and anisokaryosis. They are spindled to stellate to epithelioid (ie, may seem to cluster) with indistinct cell borders, variable amounts of basophilic cytoplasm, and a round to oval to pleomorphic nucleus (**Fig. 24**).[9,40] Variable numbers of small, punctate vacuoles are often seen in the cytoplasm.[9] Red blood cells may also be seen within the cytoplasm of neoplastic cells. Increased numbers of neutrophils (due to pooling of blood) and extramedullary hematopoiesis may be observed in both cutaneous and visceral hemangiosarcoma.[39,41] Hemangioma is better diagnosed via biopsy with histologic evaluation, as cytologic findings consist predominantly of blood and rare, morphologically unremarkable mesenchymal cells.

Melanocytic Tumors

Melanocytic tumors include benign melanocytomas and malignant melanomas (also known as melanosarcoma). These tumors are composed of melanocytes, which are cells of neural crest origin found in the basal layer of the epithelium. These neoplasms

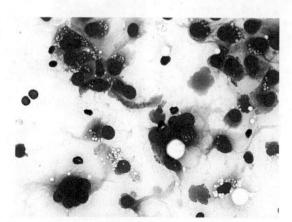

Fig. 23. Perivascular wall tumor. FNA. Dog. Cells have a moderate amount of wispy, lightly vacuolated, blue cytoplasm and a round nucleus. A crown cell containing 5 nuclei in a half-circle is present in the lower left of the image (Diff-Quik, original magnification ×60).

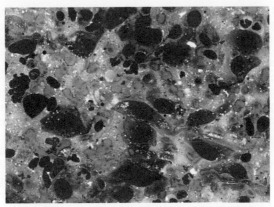

Fig. 24. Cutaneous hemangiosarcoma. FNA. Dog. Pleomorphic, neoplastic endothelial cells contain small cytoplasmic vacuoles and occasionally erythrocytes. Multiple cytologic criteria of malignancy are present. Few neutrophils are scattered throughout the image (Wright stain, original magnification ×60).

are common in dogs and less common in cats.[31] In general, melanocytic tumors associated with haired skin are more commonly benign, whereas those associated with the oral cavity or nail bed are more likely to be malignant.[31] Malignant melanomas have a high metastatic rate.[31] The gross appearance of a benign melanocytoma is typically that of a hairless, well-circumscribed, darkly pigmented nodule.[34] Malignant melanomas, on the other hand, may be variable in appearance. Pigmentation may or may not be apparent, and the mass is typically infiltrative and ulcerated.[9,34]

Melanocytoma
Cytologically, melanocytomas are moderately to highly cellular with abundant, dark green, brown, or black melanin pigment in the background. Individualized to loosely aggregated, large, round to polygonal melanocytes filled with melanin granules are the predominant cell type. The melanin granules are often abundant enough to obscure the nucleus (**Fig. 25**).[9] Individual melanin granules are appreciated on high

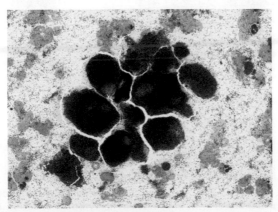

Fig. 25. Melanocytoma. FNA. Dog. Melanin granules almost entirely obscure the nucleus of these melanocytes (Wright stain, original magnification ×60).

magnification and are distinct, round to oval (rarely fusiform), green to black granules.[9] Cell size may vary significantly (marked anisocytosis); however, when nuclei can be seen through the pigment, they are uniform in size (minimal anisokaryosis).[9]

Malignant melanoma

Malignant melanoma may appear cytologically similar to a melanocytoma with the addition of increased pleomorphism and characteristics of malignancy, but they may also appear vastly different.[9] Smears of a malignant melanoma are often highly cellular and composed of cells arranged singly or in aggregates and clusters. The cells may range from round or polygonal to spindled or stellate in appearance. Cell borders are variably distinct, and nuclear to cytoplasmic ratios are also variable. Melanin granules may be present in large enough quantities to see from low magnification (similar to a melanocytoma); however, careful scrutiny on high magnification may be required to identify them, as few, fine, small melanin granules may be present (**Fig. 26**).[9] Uncommonly, melanin may be completely absent; biopsy with histopathology with special stains would be required to confirm the tissue of origin in these cases.

CUTANEOUS ROUND CELL TUMORS

The round cell tumors are grouped together because of their similar hematologic origin, shape, distinct cell borders, and arrangement as single cells rather than clusters of cells. In many cases, they can be distinguished from each other cytologically by their specific cellular features. These features are discussed next.

Cutaneous Lymphoma

Cutaneous lymphoma is most commonly a primary disease but may rarely occur in association with generalized lymphoma. The 2 forms of cutaneous lymphoma are epitheliotropic and nonepitheliotropic; the term *epitheliotropic* refers to the tendency of lymphocytes to infiltrate the epithelial layer of the skin in addition to the dermis.[9,31] Cytology does not allow for evaluation of tissue architecture, so it cannot distinguish between the 2 forms; biopsy with histologic evaluation is required for this. The gross

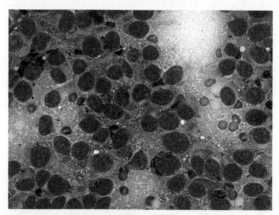

Fig. 26. Malignant melanoma. FNA. Dog. This highly cellular sample is composed of many, poorly pigmented melanocytes with high nuclear to cytoplasmic ratios. Few melanocytes contain black, granular pigment (melanin). Several cytologic criteria for malignancy are present (Diff-Quik, original magnification ×60).

appearance of these tumors is variable and ranges from patches of discolored skin (macules) to ulcers to plaques to nodules.

The cytologic findings of cutaneous lymphoma resemble those of lymphoma elsewhere in the body. Samples are typically highly cellular and composed of a uniform population of neoplastic lymphocytes, usually intermediate or large cells, in the absence or dearth of plasma cells (**Fig. 27**).[9] Lymphocyte nuclei may be round, indented, or irregular and convoluted.[9] Lymphocytes may be distinguished from other round cells by their scant amount of cytoplasm and high nuclear to cytoplasm ratio.

Mast Cell Tumor

MCTs are common and represent approximately 10% to 15% of all skin tumors in dogs and 12% to 20% of skin tumors in cats.[9,34] MCTs are particularly prevalent in boxers, Boston terriers, bull terriers, Weimaraners, and Labrador retrievers.[31] These tumors may be single or multicentric, and multiple tumors may be present in about 10% of cases.[34] MCTs have a variable gross appearance and may be white to yellow to red, alopecic and edematous masses or plaques.[31]

All canine MCTs should be treated as potentially malignant, and grading systems have been developed to determine the likelihood of metastasis. Two histologic grading systems are currently in use: one provides a grade of I, II, or III (grade III indicates a tumor with high malignant potential), whereas the other system provides a 2-tier classification of low or high malignant potential. The latter system has recently been shown to more reliably identify tumors with high malignant potential and is now the preferred histologic method.[42,43] A cytologic grading scheme for MCTs has also recently been described, and this scheme correctly identified dogs with high-grade MCTs in most cases.[44] The cytologic grading scheme is considered useful for rapidly determining prognosis and treatment options.[44] That said, grading cannot predict the biological behavior of every MCT; molecular methods may be required to obtain the most accurate prognosis.[43]

MCTs are less common in cats than dogs; but cats, particularly Siamese, have an increased tendency to develop multiple, cutaneous MCTs.[31] These tumors are typically firm, alopecic, pink to tan nodules or plaques. The previously described grading

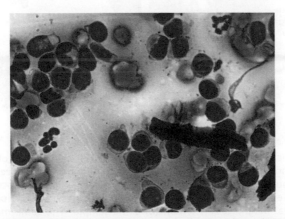

Fig. 27. Cutaneous lymphoma. FNA. Dog. Most cells in this sample are lymphocytes with few scattered neutrophils. Lymphocytes are intermediate in size (approximately the same size as a neutrophil) (Diff-Quik, original magnification ×100).

systems do not seem to correlate with prognosis in this species.[34] Fortunately, most cutaneous MCTs in cats are benign.[9,34]

Cytologically, MCTs are composed of moderate to high numbers of round (occasionally polygonal) cells that vary from poorly to highly granular. The large numbers of dark pink to purple granules may obscure the nucleus entirely (**Fig. 28**). The background will frequently contain large numbers of granules that have been released from ruptured mast cells during sample preparation. High-grade tumors frequently exhibit at least 2 of the following characteristics: presence of any mitotic figures, nuclear pleomorphism, binucleation or multi-nucleation, or marked anisokaryosis (defined as >50% variation in nuclear size).[44] Some high-grade MCTs will exhibit poor granulation as the only significant cytologic characteristic of malignancy; however, poor granulation cannot be assessed with the rapid cytologic stains typically used in a private practice setting (see the Quick tip later).[9,44,45] Unstained slides should be submitted to a clinical pathologist for accurate evaluation of cytologic grade. Other features commonly observed in canine MCTs include numerous eosinophils, proliferation of mesenchymal cells (eg, reactive fibroblasts), and fibrils of pink collagen. Eosinophils in feline MCTs tend to be sparse in numbers.

Quick tip
Mast cell granules and eosinophil granules may occasionally stain poorly with aqueous-based rapid cytologic stains (eg, Diff-Quik).[45] A mast cell that appears poorly granular or agranular with these stains may appear well granulated with methanol-based or Wright-type stains used by most reference laboratories.[45] Careful examination of a fresh cytologic specimen on high magnification is recommended to aid in the identification of mast cell granules when they are sparse and poorly stained (see **Fig. 28**).

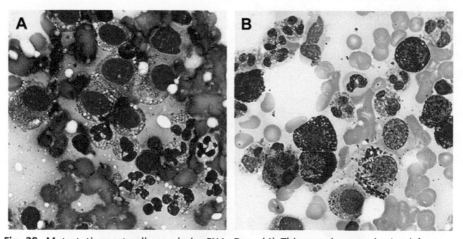

Fig. 28. Metastatic mast cell neoplasia. FNA. Dog. (*A*) This sample was obtained from an inguinal lymph node (MCT previously removed from that limb). The mast cells appear poorly granular; numerous eosinophils, one neutrophil, and few small lymphocytes are present. Eosinophil granules failed to stain, which may allow for misidentification as neutrophils (Diff-Quik, original magnification ×100). (*B*) Same sample. The same mast cells as in A contain more abundant, purple granules that nearly obscure the nucleus. Few mast cells still appear poorly granular. Eosinophil granules stained pink. A single small lymphocyte and neutrophil are present in this image (Wright stain, original magnification ×100).

Cutaneous Plasmacytoma

Cutaneous plasmacytomas represent 1.5% to 2.0% of skin tumors in dogs and are typically benign.[34] Cats are rarely affected.[34] These tumors tend to occur on the digits, ears, and mouth and are typically firm, well-circumscribed, alopecic, dermal nodules.[9]

Cytologic examination of these tumors reveals a highly cellular sample composed of oval cells with distinct borders. These cells contain a variable amount of basophilic cytoplasm and an eccentrically placed nucleus. Often, there is a clearing or pale area of the cytoplasm adjacent to the nucleus (**Fig. 29**). The nucleus of a plasma cell typically contains patchy, clumped chromatin. Despite the often benign behavior of these tumors, they can display strong cytologic characteristics of malignancy such as marked anisocytosis and anisokaryosis, binucleation, and multi-nucleation (**Fig. 30**).[9,34,46]

Cutaneous Histiocytoma

Cutaneous histiocytoma is a very common, benign tumor of the head, ears, neck, or legs of young dogs.[9,34] Dogs greater than 3 years of age are uncommonly affected.[34] The classic appearance of the tumor is that of a small, red, dome-shaped, smooth and alopecic nodule sometimes described as button-like.[31] These tumors usually spontaneously regress after a short time and do not cause clinically significant disease unless they become ulcerated and secondarily infected.[31]

Cytologic evaluation reveals high cellularity with numerous round to oval cells in a hazy, blue, proteinaceous background (**Fig. 31**). These cells are about 1.0 to 1.5 times the size of a neutrophil with distinct cell borders and smooth, pale blue, generally non-vacuolated cytoplasm. The nucleus is typically oval to bean shaped and centrally to eccentrically located. The cells are uniform in appearance with minimal cytologic characteristics of malignancy.[9] Variable numbers of small lymphocytes may be admixed with the neoplastic cells, especially when the tumor is in the process of regressing.[9]

Histiocytic Sarcoma

This neoplasm may be primarily localized in the subcutaneous tissues or it may be disseminated. The disseminated form was previously referred to as malignant

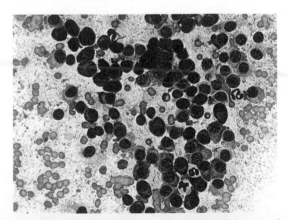

Fig. 29. Cutaneous plasma cell tumor. FNA. Cat. This highly cellular sample is composed predominantly of neoplastic plasma cells with few neutrophils. Plasma cells exhibit occasional binucleation and mildly variable nuclear to cytoplasmic ratios (Wright stain, original magnification ×60).

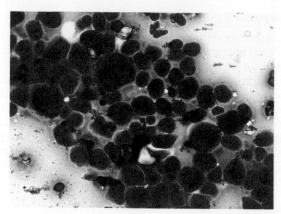

Fig. 30. Cutaneous plasma cell tumor. FNA. Dog. Neoplastic plasma cells exhibit bizarre features, such as multi-nucleation and anisokaryosis, despite the benign nature of this tumor (Diff-Quik, original magnification ×60).

histiocytosis.[34] The localized, subcutaneous form of histiocytic sarcoma is fairly common in dogs, particularly in Bernese mountain dogs, Rottweilers, and golden and Labrador retrievers, but is rare in cats.[34] These neoplasms are typically firm, variably sized, subcutaneous masses that may become quite large and invasive.[34] The localized form is most often identified on extremities, particularly around joints, whereas the disseminated form may result in cutaneous masses anywhere on the body in addition to internal lesions.[34]

Cytologic findings may be highly variable for this neoplasm. The cells typically have a discrete, round cell appearance; but they may also have a slightly spindled appearance.[9] Cells often contain abundant, blue cytoplasm that may be vacuolated.[9] A key feature of this neoplasm is the malignant cytologic appearance, characterized by marked anisocytosis and anisokaryosis, bizarre nuclear shapes, karyomegaly, binucleation and multinucleation, and atypical mitotic figures (**Fig. 32**).[35]

This neoplasm is often difficult to distinguish cytologically from other malignant tumors, such as amelanotic melanomas, anaplastic sarcomas with giant cells, plasma

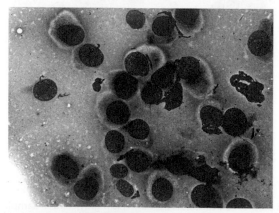

Fig. 31. Cutaneous histiocytoma. FNA. Dog. Round to oval histiocytes are arranged as single cells in a characteristic, hazy, blue background. They are relatively uniform in size with no obvious cytologic characteristics of malignancy (Diff-Quik, original magnification ×100).

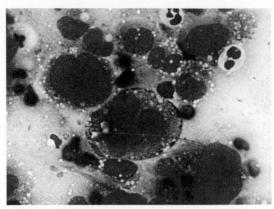

Fig. 32. Histiocytic sarcoma. FNA. Dog. These neoplastic histiocytes are markedly pleomorphic and exhibit numerous cytologic characteristics of malignancy. Two neutrophils and a small lymphocyte are also present (Diff-Quik, original magnification ×100).

cell tumors, and poorly differentiated MCTs. Biopsy and histologic examination with special stains is often required for a confident diagnosis.[9]

Transmissible Venereal Tumor

Transmissible venereal tumor (TVT) is only reported in canids and is one of the few reported tumors that may be transmitted via direct physical transplantation of neoplastic cells from one host to another.[31] This neoplasm occurs in a patchy distribution around the world and is common in some regions of the Caribbean.[31] Veterinary practitioners should consider TVT when encountering a sexually active dog with a red, fleshy, multinodular, poorly circumscribed mass associated with the genitalia or mucous membranes of the face.[9] TVT can also be present in neutered or spayed dogs as a result of the sniffing social behavior in this species.

Cytologically, these neoplasms are highly cellular and exhibit excellent exfoliation with FNA or direct imprint of the mass onto a glass slide.[9] Neoplastic cells are 1.0 to 1.5 times the size of a neutrophil and are round, individualized cells with distinct

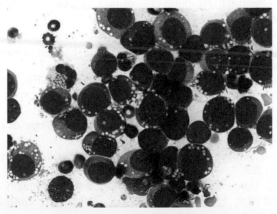

Fig. 33. TVT. FNA. Dog. The distinct cytoplasmic vacuoles are a key feature of this neoplasm. This particular tumor was ulcerated and secondarily infected, as evidenced by the bacterial rods within neutrophils and in the background (Diff-Quik, original magnification ×100).

cell borders. They contain a moderate amount of light to medium blue cytoplasm with several, clear, punctate, intracytoplasmic vacuoles. These vacuoles are a key feature and often help to differentiate TVT from other round cell tumors **(Fig. 33)**.[34] The cells contain a single, round nucleus with one or 2 prominent nucleoli. Mitotic figures may be numerous.

SUMMARY

Although not a replacement for excisional biopsy and histologic evaluation, cytology is a viable diagnostic modality to provide both general and specific diagnostic information for treatment considerations of skin masses in dogs and cats. Using key cytologic features addressed in these sections, veterinarians should be able to differentiate and identify various types of skin neoplasms encountered in their patients. This skill should allow veterinarians the ability to make appropriate recommendations to their clients in regard to treatment options and further diagnostic considerations.

REFERENCES

1. Meinkoth JH, Cowell RL, Tyler RD. Cell types and criteria of malignancy. In: Valenciano AC, Cowell RL, editors. Diagnostic cytology and hematology of the dog and cat. 4th edition. St Louis (MO): Elsevier Mosby; 2013. p. 20–47.
2. Clifford CA, de Lorimier LP, Fan TM, et al. Neoplastic and non-neoplastic tumors. In: Miller WH, Griffin CE, Campbell KL, editors. Muller & Kirk's small animal dermatology. 7th edition. St Louis (MO): Elsevier Mosby; 2013. p. 774–843.
3. White A, Stern A, Campbell K, et al. Multiple (disseminated) follicular cysts in five dogs and one cat. Vet Rec 2013;173(11):269.
4. Tyler RD, Cowell RL, Meinkoth JH. Cutaneous and subcutaneous lesions. In: Cowell RL, Tyler RD, Meinkoth JH, et al, editors. Diagnostic cytology and hematology of the dog and cat. 3rd edition. St Louis (MO): Mosby Elsevier; 2008. p. 78–111.
5. Goldschmidt MH, Thrall DE, Jeglum KA, et al. Malignant pilomatricoma in a dog. J Cutan Pathol 1981;8(5):375–81.
6. Carroll EE, Fossey SL, Mangus LM, et al. Malignant pilomatricoma in 3 dogs. Vet Pathol 2010;47(5):937–43.
7. da Silva EO, Green KT, Wasques DG, et al. Malignant pilomatricoma in a dog. J Comp Pathol 2012;147(2–3):214–7.
8. Barrot AC, Carioto L, Gains M, et al. Metastatic malignant pilomatrixoma, acanthomatous ameloblastoma, and liver tumor in a dog with polyphagia, polyuria, polydipsia, and weight loss. Can Vet J 2013;54(4):387–91.
9. Raskin RE. Skin and subcutaneous tissues. In: Raskin RE, Meyer DJ, editors. Canine and feline cytology: a color atlas and interpretation guide. 3rd edition. St Louis (MO): Elsevier; 2016. p. 34–90.
10. Masserdotti C, Ubbiali FA. Fine needle aspiration cytology of pilomatricoma in three dogs. Vet Clin Pathol 2002;31(1):22–5.
11. Watt FM, Jensen KB. Epidermal stem cell diversity and quiescence. EMBO Mol Med 2009;1(5):260–7.
12. Brachelente C, Porcellato I, Sforna M, et al. The contribution of stem cells to epidermal and hair follicle tumours in the dog. Vet Dermatol 2013;24(1):188–94.e41.
13. Quist SR, Eckardt M, Kriesche A, et al. Expression of stem cell markers in skin and adnexal malignancies. Br J Dermatol 2016. [Epub ahead of print].

14. Pisani G, Millanta F, Lorenzi D, et al. Androgen receptor expression in normal, hyperplastic and neoplastic hepatoid glands in the dog. Res Vet Sci 2006;81(2):231–6.
15. Martins AM, Vasques-Peyser A, Torres LN, et al. Retrospective–systematic study and quantitative analysis of cellular proliferation and apoptosis in normal, hyperplastic and neoplastic perianal glands in dogs. Vet Comp Oncol 2008;6(2):71–9.
16. Javanbakht J, Tavassoli A, Sasani F, et al. An overall assessment of circumanal gland adenoma in a terrier mix breed dog. Asian Pac J Trop Biomed 2013;3(7):580–3.
17. Rosol TJ, Nagode LA, Couto CG, et al. Parathyroid hormone (PTH)-related protein, PTH, and 1,25-dihydroxyvitamin D in dogs with cancer-associated hypercalcemia. Endocrinology 1992;131(3):1157–64.
18. Bergman PJ. Paraneoplastic hypercalcemia. Top Companion Anim Med 2012;27(4):156–8.
19. Petterino C, Woodger N. What is your diagnosis? Perianal gland mass in a cat. Anal sac gland carcinoma. Vet Clin Pathol 2014;43(4):611–2.
20. Moisan PG, Watson GL. Ceruminous gland tumors in dogs and cats: a review of 124 cases. J Am Anim Hosp Assoc 1996;32(5):448–52.
21. De Lorenzi D, Bonfanti U, Masserdotti C, et al. Fine-needle biopsy of external ear canal masses in the cat: cytologic results and histologic correlations in 27 cases. Vet Clin Pathol 2005;34(2):100–5.
22. Gross TL, Ihrke PJ, Walder EJ, et al. Epithelial neoplasms and other tumors. In: Skin diseases of the dog and cat: clinical and histopathologic diagnosis. Oxford (United Kingdom): Blackwell Science Ltd; 2005. p. 561–708.
23. Simko E, Wilcock BP, Yager JA. A retrospective study of 44 canine apocrine sweat gland adenocarcinomas. Can Vet J 2003;44(1):38–42.
24. Munday JS, Hanlon EM, Howe L, et al. Feline cutaneous viral papilloma associated with human papillomavirus type 9. Vet Pathol 2007;44(6):924–7.
25. Egberink H, Thiry E, Mostl K, et al. Feline viral papillomatosis: ABCD guidelines on prevention and management. J Feline Med Surg 2013;15(7):560–2.
26. Teifke JP, Lohr CV, Shirasawa H. Detection of canine oral papillomavirus-DNA in canine oral squamous cell carcinomas and p53 overexpressing skin papillomas of the dog using the polymerase chain reaction and non-radioactive in situ hybridization. Vet Microbiol 1998;60(2–4):119–30.
27. Debey BM, Bagladi-Swanson M, Kapil S, et al. Digital papillomatosis in a confined beagle. J Vet Diagn Invest 2001;13(4):346–8.
28. Lange CE, Tobler K, Brandes K, et al. Canine inverted papillomas associated with DNA of four different papillomaviruses. Vet Dermatol 2010;21(3):287–91.
29. Beckwith-Cohen B, Teixeira LB, Ramos-Vara JA, et al. Squamous papillomas of the conjunctiva in dogs: a condition not associated with papillomavirus infection. Vet Pathol 2015;52(4):676–80.
30. Wiggans KT, Hoover CE, Ehrhart EJ, et al. Malignant transformation of a putative eyelid papilloma to squamous cell carcinoma in a dog. Vet Ophthalmol 2013;16(Suppl 1):105–12.
31. Goldschmidt MH, Hendrick MJ. Tumors of the skin and soft tissues. In: Meuten DJ, editor. Tumors in domestic animals. 4th edition. Ames (IA): Iowa State Press; 2003. p. 45–117.
32. Liptak JM, Forrest LJ. Soft tissue sarcomas. In: Withrow SJ, Vail DM, Page RL, editors. Withrow and MacEwen's small animal clinical oncology. 5th edition. St Louis (MO): Elsevier Saunders; 2013. p. 356–80.

33. Hohenhaus AE, Kelsey JL, Haddad J, et al. Canine cutaneous and subcutaneous soft tissue sarcoma: an evidence-based review of case management. J Am Anim Hosp Assoc 2016;52(2):77–89.

34. Gross TL, Ihrke PJ, Walder EJ, et al. Mesenchymal neoplasms and other tumors. In: Skin diseases of the dog and cat: clinical and histopathologic diagnosis. 2nd edition. Oxford (United Kingdom): Blackwell Science Ltd; 2005. p. 709–894.

35. Fisher DJ. Cutaneous and subcutaneous lesions. In: Valenciano AC, Cowell RL, editors. Cowell and Tyler's diagnostic cytology and hematology of the dog and cat. 4th edition. St Louis (MO): Elsevier Mosby; 2013. p. 80–109.

36. Avallone G, Helmbold P, Caniatti M, et al. The spectrum of canine cutaneous perivascular wall tumors: morphologic, phenotypic and clinical characterization. Vet Pathol 2007;44(5):607–20.

37. Hargis AM, Ihrke PJ, Spangler WL, et al. A retrospective clinicopathologic study of 212 dogs with cutaneous hemangiomas and hemangiosarcomas. Vet Pathol 1992;29(4):316–28.

38. Ward H, Fox LE, Calderwood-Mays MB, et al. Cutaneous hemangiosarcoma in 25 dogs: a retrospective study. J Vet Intern Med 1994;8(5):345–8.

39. Bertazzolo W, Dell'Orco M, Bonfanti U, et al. Canine angiosarcoma: cytologic, histologic, and immunohistochemical correlations. Vet Clin Pathol 2005;34(1):28–34.

40. Wilkerson MJ, Chard-Bergstrom C, Andrews G, et al. Subcutaneous mass aspirate from a dog. Vet Clin Pathol 2002;31(2):65–8.

41. Dunbar MD, Conway JA. What is your diagnosis? Cytologic findings from a subcutaneous nodule over the left epaxial musculature in a dog. Vet Clin Pathol 2012; 41(2):295–6.

42. Kiupel M, Webster JD, Bailey KL, et al. Proposal of a 2-tier histologic grading system for canine cutaneous mast cell tumors to more accurately predict biological behavior. Vet Pathol 2011;48(1):147–55.

43. Sabattini S, Scarpa F, Berlato D, et al. Histologic grading of canine mast cell tumor: is 2 better than 3? Vet Pathol 2015;52(1):70–3.

44. Camus MS, Priest HL, Koehler JW, et al. Cytologic criteria for mast cell tumor grading in dogs with evaluation of clinical outcome. Vet Pathol 2016. [Epub ahead of print].

45. Leclere M, Desnoyers M, Beauchamp G, et al. Comparison of four staining methods for detection of mast cells in equine bronchoalveolar lavage fluid. J Vet Intern Med 2006;20(2):377–81.

46. Baer KE, Patnaik AK, Gilbertson SR, et al. Cutaneous plasmacytomas in dogs: a morphologic and immunohistochemical study. Vet Pathol 1989;26(3):216–21.

Preanalytical Considerations for Joint Fluid Evaluation

Caitlyn R. Martinez, DVM, Kelly S. Santangelo, DVM, PhD*

KEYWORDS

- Synovial fluid • Orthopedics • Osteoarthritis • Immune-mediated polyarthropathy
- Septic arthritis

KEY POINTS

- Synovial fluid analysis is a key component of the minimum database needed to diagnose and manage primary and secondary articular joint disorders.
- Preanalytical variables can drastically alter samples submitted to veterinary laboratories for evaluation and it is considered the stage at which most laboratory error occurs.
- Common indications for the collection of synovial fluid include orthopedic lameness; abnormal limb function or gait; articular pain and/or distention; fever of unknown origin; or widespread pain, stiffness, or difficulty moving.
- The gross characteristics of synovial fluid yield important information as to the quality and pathology of the joint and should be noted at the time of sample collection.
- When arthrocentesis yields small sample volumes, cytologic evaluation of direct smears offers the most clinically relevant information available from synovial fluid.

INTRODUCTION

In concert with clinical history, physical examination, imaging modalities, and other clinical pathology findings, synovial fluid analysis is a key component of the minimum database needed to diagnose and manage primary and secondary articular joint disorders. The preanalytical phase of synovial fluid evaluation encompasses the steps from initial sample collection through final arrival and accessioning at the diagnostic laboratory. Unfortunately, preanalytical variables can drastically alter samples submitted for evaluation to veterinary laboratories and it is considered the stage at which most laboratory error occurs.[1] Specific variables that may influence the interpretation

The authors have nothing to disclose.
Department of Microbiology, Immunology, and Pathology, College of Veterinary Medicine and Biomedical Sciences, Colorado State University, 1644 Campus Delivery, Fort Collins, CO 80523, USA
* Corresponding author.
E-mail address: kelly.santangelo@colostate.edu

Vet Clin Small Anim 47 (2017) 111–122
http://dx.doi.org/10.1016/j.cvsm.2016.07.007
vetsmall.theclinics.com

of joint fluid mostly involve technical factors, such as selection of collection materials, evidence of blood contamination, and specimen handling. Other considerations that should be included with sample submission include the location that was aspirated, the signalment and presenting signs of the animal, and current medications being administered. With consistent preanalytical quality control and reporting of specimens, downstream clinical decision making and management of patients can be accelerated and improved. General practitioners should always feel comfortable contacting a diagnostic laboratory for specific information regarding sample acquisition, processing, and submission.[2,3]

ORIGINS AND CHARACTERISTICS OF SYNOVIAL FLUID

Joints are the points of interaction and movement between 2 adjacent bones. Hyaline cartilage overlays the subchondral bone and is the contact surface. Chondrocytes within the articular cartilage produce the proteoglycans present in the cartilage. This articular space is enclosed by a joint capsule. The joint capsule is composed of a tough, fibrous external surface, a vascular subsynovial layer, and the lining synovial surface. The synovium is thin and contains 2 types of cells, or synoviocytes. These cells are either phagocytic and thus similar to macrophages (type A synoviocytes), or they produce hyaluronic acid, a glycosaminoglycan (type B synoviocytes).[4] Both types of synoviocytes can be visualized on cytologic preparations of synovial fluid, but are typically difficult to differentiate in normal joints and are classified together as large mononuclear cells.

Synovial fluid from a nondiseased joint is an ultrafiltrate of plasma that is modified by secretion of hyaluronic acid, glycoproteins, and other macromolecules. Smaller molecules, such as glucose and electrolytes, can occur in synovial fluid in concentrations equivalent to those in plasma. Proteins from plasma, however, are included in this synovial dialysate only to a limited extent. Synovial fluid serves 2 major purposes. First, it provides a source of nutrition and waste removal from articular chondrocytes. Second, joint fluid lubricates opposing articular cartilage surfaces, limiting friction and wear during contact. Although hyaluronic acid has some lubricating properties, glycoproteins are the primary source of reduced friction during joint motion.

When the components of the joint become diseased, injured, and/or inflamed, pathology is frequently reflected by changes within synovial fluid. Evidence of abnormal conditions include joint effusion with decreased viscosity and increased protein content, increased numbers of inflammatory cells, changes in the percentages of different cell types present, and intra-articular hemorrhage.

INDICATIONS FOR COLLECTION OF SYNOVIAL FLUID

Synovial fluid analysis is a critical aspect of the workup for an animal exhibiting joint issues, whether these concerns are primary maladies localized to one or more limbs or reflect the secondary manifestation of a systemic condition. Importantly, these data must be integrated with other clinical and laboratory findings, including culture, serology, antinuclear antibody titer, and rheumatoid factor titer. Common indications for the collection of synovial fluid include orthopedic lameness, abnormal limb function or gait, articular pain and/or distention; fever of unknown origin; or widespread pain, stiffness, or difficulty moving.[5]

Typical characteristics of synovial fluid from dogs and cats are presented in **Table 1**. Normal synovial fluid is light yellow and clear, with no observable particular material. The volume that can be aspirated depends on the joint being sampled and the condition of the joint. For most large breed dogs, less than 0.5 mL of synovial fluid is

Table 1				
Normal synovial fluid characteristics in dogs and cats				
Species	**TNCC (Cells/µL)**	**% Neutrophils**	**Expected Volume, mL**	**Gross Appearance**
Dog	≤2900	≤12	≤0.5	Light yellow
Cat	≤1134	≤39	≤0.25	Clear
				Highly viscous
				Thixotropic

Abbreviation: TNCC, total nucleated cell count.
  Data from Refs.[11,18,19,37]

expected from most joints. Up to 1 mL of fluid can be collected from stifle joints,[6] and the volume of joint fluid obtained from dogs with hip dysplasia can range from 2 to 6 mL.[7] Joints from small dogs and cats do not typically yield more than 0.25 mL of synovial fluid.

RECOMMENDATIONS FOR SAMPLE COLLECTION
Collection Sites

Routine sterile technique should be followed for all arthrocentesis procedures, including the clipping of fur and thorough scrubbing of the area. The clinician should judge the amount of restraint and sedation or anesthesia needed to accomplish joint fluid collection in the absence of complications. Ultrasonography is frequently used and recommended for guiding arthrocentesis procedures and characterizing joint lesions in humans.[8,9] Unwanted events include blood contamination, retrieving an insufficient volume of synovial fluid, scratching articular surfaces, or damaging local blood vessels, nerves, or the synovial membrane. Before removing the needle from the joint, the plunger of the syringe should be released to eliminate negative pressure.

Brief descriptions of recommended approaches to synovial fluid collection from articular joints are provided in **Table 2**. When noninfectious polyarthritis is a differential diagnosis, it is recommended that arthrocentesis be performed on multiple joints, specifically the carpi, tarsi, and stifle joints. Clinical signs commonly associated with polyarthritis include leg-shifting lameness, fever of unknown origin, and joint pain. Of note, however, one retrospective study documented that polyarthritis also can present simply as difficulty walking, without any other significant findings.[10]

Collection Materials

Needles and syringes
Sterile disposable 0.75-inch to 1-inch, 22-gauge or 25-gauge hypodermic needles connected to 3-mL to 6-mL syringes are recommended. Some researchers prefer a 25-gauge needle attached to a 1-mL or 3-mL syringe for feline arthrocentesis, as increased blood contamination is noted with larger-bore needles.[11] In larger-breed dogs, sampling of the shoulder or elbow joint may necessitate a 1.5-inch needle, whereas the hip may require a 3.0-inch spinal needle.

Tube selection
When inflamed synovial membranes have increased vascular permeability, this allows increased proteins, such as fibrinogen, into joint fluid. This often results in clotting of synovial fluid samples. Clotting can also occur with significant hemorrhage or blood contamination. Given this, it is recommended to aliquot a portion of the sample into an ethylenediaminetetraacetic acid (EDTA) tube to prevent coagulation and allow for additional analyses.[5] The smallest EDTA blood tube available should be used to avoid

Table 2
Suggested positioning and entry for arthrocentesis of common joints

Articular Joint	Position	Needle Entry	Needle Advancement
Stifle	Flexed	Lateral to patellar tendon and distal to patella	Needle is advanced in a medial and proximal direction, pointing toward the medial condyle of the femur
Hip	Femur is abducted and leg extended caudally	Cranial to the greater trochanter of the femur	Needle is inserted caudal and distal to the joint
Shoulder	Neutral to flexed	Distal to the acromion of the scapula and caudal to the greater tubercles of the humerus	Needle is directed medially toward the greater tubercle and just distal to the supraglenoid tubercle of the scapula
Elbow	Extended or flexed	Extended: Medial to the lateral epicondyle of the humerus and lateral to the olecranon Flexed: Proximal to the olecranon and medial to the lateral epicondylar crest	Needle is inserted parallel to the olecranon and the long axis of the ulna
Carpus	Flexed	Antebrachiocarpal joint: Between the distal radius and proximal radial carpal bone Middle carpal joint: Distal portion of the radial carpal bone and the second and third carpal bones	Needle is introduced from the dorsal aspect, just medial of center, and inserted perpendicular to joint
Tarsus	Extended or flexed	Extended (caudal approach): Medial or lateral to the calcaneus Flexed (cranial approach): Space palpated between tibia and talus bones, just lateral to the tendon bundle	Extended: Needle is advanced with a cranial and slightly plantar path Flexed: Needle is inserted perpendicular to palpated space

erroneous results due to sample dilution from excess anticoagulant. If small tubes are not available, then excess EDTA can be decanted from the vessel before adding the sample.

In contrast, EDTA can cause disruption of hyaluronic acid. Therefore, it is not recommended to evaluate synovial fluid viscosity or mucin clot formation from EDTA samples. When this is desired, sample should be provided in a tube that does not contain this particular anticoagulant, such as a red top tube or a heparin tube.[12]

For samples that are to be cultured, fluid should be left in the sterile syringe and/or placed into an aerobic culturette or blood culture tube. A red top tube also may be used for this purpose if sterility can be maintained. To increase the likelihood of a positive culture, it is recommended to place the synovial fluid sample in blood culture media if available. Synovial membrane biopsy for culture is not recommended, as it has been shown to be less successful at yielding positive culture results than synovial fluid culture. Additionally, synovial membrane biopsy is considerably more invasive and traumatic than arthrocentesis.[13]

Sequential Arthrocentesis

Sequential arthrocentesis and synovial fluid analysis is often performed as part of the therapeutic monitoring of immune-mediated polyarthritis. It is recognized that arthrocentesis is a traumatic procedure and may elicit mild mononuclear inflammation. However, one study performed in healthy dogs showed that synovial fluid collection every 3 weeks did not result in differing cell counts or percentages.[14] Thus, repeated collections using this length of time are considered less likely to be clinically significant or obscure evidence of a therapeutic response.

VISUAL ASSESSMENT OF COLLECTED SAMPLE

The gross characteristics of synovial fluid yield important information as to the quality and pathology of the joint and should be noted at the time of sample collection. Even when limited sample is available and only a direct smear can be prepared, it is still possible to evaluate the approximate volume, color, viscosity, and turbidity of synovial fluid as the sample is aspirated, expelled onto a slide, and smeared.[15] Homogeneously red or red-tinged fluid indicates hemorrhage in the joint, which is usually associated with trauma or inflammation. This should be differentiated from blood contamination, as discussed later in this article. Xanthochromia, which imparts a yellow-orange discoloration to joint fluid due to hemoglobin breakdown, may be seen following the resolution of hemorrhage. Overt sediment and/or white or light yellow coloration indicates either an increase in the nucleated cell count, usually due to inflammation, infection, or neoplasia, or the presence of crystals. Increased turbidity results from suspended particulate matter, which may be related to red or white cells, fibrin, bacteria/organisms, or, less commonly, crystals. It is rare for crystals or neoplastic cells, alone, to cause changes in color or turbidity.[16]

It is important to recognize that normal synovial fluid does not clot in a tube or syringe, but instead forms a gel. Distinction of these 2 states can be accomplished by agitation of the sample, which will cause the gel, but not a clot, to return to its fluid state. This reversible fluid-gel phenomenon is called thixotropism.

VALUE OF DIRECT SMEAR PREPARATION

Small animal arthrocentesis often yields limited sample volume. In such scenarios, it is commonly advised that cytologic evaluation of direct smears offers the most clinically relevant information available from synovial fluid.[15,17,18] Given the viscosity of joint fluid, a squash or compression preparation is typically used to generate direct smears. It is recommended that direct smears be made immediately following sample collection and before any additional processing. This prevents artifacts or misinterpretations due to sample aging, concentration, dilution, or contamination.[2,3] A rough estimation of total nucleated cell count (TNCC), differential counts, characterization of any unusual cells that may be present, as well as a subjective assessment of the proteoglycan background, are all possible to evaluate from a direct smear, alone. Indeed, direct smears are often preferred over cytocentrifuge-prepared slides for differential cell counts, as some researchers feel that the latter may not provide an accurate representation of cell proportions and that the morphology of the cells may be altered during centrifugation.[2,19] In particular, a diagnosis of suppurative inflammation can be reliably made using direct smears.[20] If sample quantity allows, recommended additional tests include TNCC (obtained via automated or hemocytometer methods), total protein, and mucin clot test. If there is concern for bacterial arthritis, 2 to 3 drops of synovial fluid for culture and sensitivity can be placed into a culturette.

One issue with direct smears is that highly viscous synovial fluid often yields thick preparations with cell clumping and severely rounded up cells that cannot be easily identified or counted. This tends not to be a problem, however, when the joint is diseased and the synovial fluid is dilute. To address thick samples, hyaluronidase can be added to synovial fluid before slide preparation. It is recommended that 150 IU/mL hyaluronidase be mixed with an equal volume of joint fluid and incubated for several minutes before direct smear slide preparation.[19] When used, it is suggested to use gentle smearing technique, as the hyaluronidase treatment tends to cause the cells to become more fragile.

Direct smears should always be evaluated before submission to ensure adequate cellularity and distribution of synovial fluid. However, certain caveats should be emphasized, even to pathologists. First, it has been shown that the estimation of total cell count on direct smears varies from clinician to clinician and can often overestimate true cell numbers.[20] Further, distinguishing between normal synovial fluid and synovial fluid reflective of degenerative joint disease or osteoarthritis is not consistent using direct smears. Finally, direct smears should not be used as the sole indication of disease progression or evidence for therapeutic efficacy.[20]

KEY INFORMATION TO PROVIDE WITH SAMPLE SUBMISSION
Signalment

The species, age, breed, and gender of an animal can provide key information for prioritizing potential diagnoses. For example, synovial cell sarcoma is a rare tumor in animals, but occurs far more commonly in dogs than cats.[21] Clinical signs of polyarthritis syndrome in akitas typically appear before 8 months of age.[22] Bernese mountain dogs have the highest prevalence for the systemic form of histiocytic sarcoma; however, skeletal manifestation of this disease occur far more commonly in rottweilers and golden retrievers.[23]

Pertinent Clinical History

Patient history can help characterize the disease process and narrow the differential list. For example, bacterial septic arthritis may develop following articular surgery, local trauma and direct inoculation, extension from regional infections, or hematogenous spread.[24] In one case, septic arthritis occurred secondary to a migrating porcupine quill, which had been reported to travel 10 inches under the skin.[25] Bacterial septic arthritis is often thought to present as acute, severe lameness but it may also develop as chronic, mild pain without significant orthopedic impairment.[26] Immune-mediated polyarthropathy has been associated with a variety of processes, such as vaccine reactions, drug reactions, existing neoplasia, gastrointestinal disease, and idiopathic causes.[27] Suspicion for foreign body reactions, with or without secondary infection, also relies on a complete discussion of pertinent events, even if these events are not recent. For instance, onset of severe arthropathy was reported in a dog 21 months after being shot in the elbow with a lead bullet.[28] Interestingly, the metallic fragments did not mechanically interfere with joint motion.

Location(s) Aspirated

Noting the joints affected and the joints aspirated can help delineate the full extent of disease and place emphasis on one diagnosis over another. For instance, the inflammation associated with immune-mediated polyarthropathy is thought to be elicited by complement activation following antigen-antibody complex deposition within the synovium of multiple joints. Of note, lesions are most commonly observed in smaller joints, such as the carpi and tarsi.[29]

Current Medications and Nutritional Supplements

Administration of any medication should be provided on the submission form, especially if that treatment is directed at a disorder on the differential list. This includes systemic medications, as well as local, regional, and topical drugs. Of note, it is well-demonstrated that the application of nonsteroidal anti-inflammatory drugs on the skin can penetrate local tissues into the synovial fluid.[30]

It also may be pertinent to disclose the use of nutraceuticals and other supplements. Clinical trials that support the use of glucosamine, chondroitin sulfate, P54FP (a turmeric extract), omega-3 fatty acids, *Boswellia serrata* (a tree extract), and avocado-soybean unsaponifiable extracts in dogs with osteoarthritis, after surgery or trauma, and for prophylactic measures have been reported.[31] However, these studies are limited in number and there remains a need for additional randomized controlled clinical trials. Further, despite the perception that joint health products are safe based on high LD50 values and an absence of persistent adverse effects, veterinarians should be aware that contamination issues, including toxins, pesticides, and heavy metals, and metabolic concerns, particularly the use of glucosamine in individuals with type 2 diabetes, are being addressed in human and animal studies.[31]

Blood Contamination

Careful observation during arthrocentesis may demonstrate a flash of blood in the sample, indicative of blood contamination. Alternatively, a diffusely bloody sample may indicate that the sample is associated with true hemorrhage. As these separate scenarios may appear similar following shipment and arrival to the laboratory, it is important that differentiation of the 2 be documented during sample submission.[5]

SHIPPING RECOMMENDATIONS

Synovial fluid supplied in tubes or syringes can be stored or shipped at 4°C for up to 24 hours without significant loss of cytologic integrity. Therefore, it is recommended that samples being sent to laboratories be packaged with cold packs and shipped overnight to maintain sample value.[32] When providing direct smears, ensure that these slides are completely dry before packaging and kept away from exposure to formalin fumes. Do not refrigerate slides, as subsequent condensation may result in cell lysis.

DIFFERENTIAL DIAGNOSES

Several excellent textbook and review articles are available that discuss approaches to the analytical phase of synovial fluid evaluation. This stage includes cytologic evaluation of the sample, as well as a description of its appearance, protein content, viscosity, mucin clot test, nucleated cell count, and differential. In particular, the reader is referred to a wonderfully thorough article by MacWilliams and Fredericks, published by this compendium in 2003.[16]

Briefly, during the analytical phase of cytologic examination, cells will be differentially counted as small mononuclear, large mononuclear, or neutrophils. Cells will be further characterized by nuclear morphology (such as degeneration in neutrophils) and degree of vacuolization (an indication of activation in macrophages), as well as any other significant features.[29] Other cells that may be present will be described and interpreted. The sample will be carefully screened for the presence of any infectious agents. Cells are typically found on an eosinophilic, finely granular background

Table 3
Three general categories of arthropathies in veterinary medicine and associated differential diagnoses

Hemarthrosis	Noninflammatory Arthropathy
Red to xanthochromic appearance with increased protein, decreased viscosity, and normal to poor mucin clot. TNCC will be increased in proportion to the amount of blood. May see hemosiderin, hematoidin, and erythrophagia.[19,29,38]	Clear appearance with normal to decreased protein and viscosity, normal to poor mucin clot. TNCC will be normal to moderately increased with ≥90% small and large mononuclear cells. Cells may have increased vacuolization.[29,38]
Coagulopathy	Degenerative joint disease
Joint trauma	Joint trauma (ie, cranial cruciate ligament rupture)
Some neoplasms	Some neoplasms

Inflammatory Arthropathy

Cloudy appearance with normal to increased protein, normal to decreased viscosity, and fair to poor mucin clot. TNCC will be mildly to markedly increased with >10%–100% neutrophils.[38] Some specific processes may be predominantly mononuclear or eosinophilic inflammation rather than suppurative.

Infectious	Erosive	Nonerosive	Others
May see degenerate neutrophils. May see infectious organisms. Monoarticular or polyarticular.	Radiographic evidence of articular erosion. Frequently polyarticular.	Erosive and infectious disease have been ruled out. Frequently polyarticular.	May see neoplastic cells or crystals on cytology. Frequently induce an inflammatory response.
Bacteria (cocci, rods, L-forms)[24–26,39] Fungi (Coccidioides, Aspergillus, Histoplasma, Blastomyces, Cryptococcus)[40–44] Rickettsia/Ehrlichia spp.[34–36] Borrelia burgdorferi[27,45] Mycoplasma spp[46,47] Leishmania spp[48] West Nile virus (dog)[49] Feline calcivirus[50,51] Feline coronavirus (FIP)[52] Canine distemper virus[53]	Rheumatoid arthritis[54] Greyhound erosive polyarthritis[55] Juvenile-onset polyarthritis syndrome in akitas[22] Shar pei fever[56] Chronic progressive polyarthritis (cat)[57,58]	Systemic lupus erythematosus[27] Idiopathic polyarthritis[27] Idiopathic localized eosinophilic arthritis (cat)[59] Drug-induced polyarthritis[60] Lymphoplasmacytic synovitis[61] Postvaccinal arthritis[27,62] Polyarthritis polymyositis syndrome[63]	Joint trauma[28] Neoplasia Primary Histiocytic sarcoma[23,64–67] Synovial cell sarcoma[21,67,68] Synovial myxoma[67] Malignant fibrous histiocytoma[67] Fibrosarcoma[67] Chondrosarcoma[67] Undifferentiated sarcoma[67] Benign giant cell tumor of the tendon sheath[69] Lymphoma[70] Osteosarcoma[71] Hemangioma[72] Metastatic Transitional cell carcinoma[73] Mammary adenocarcinoma[74] Bronchiolar-alveolar carcinoma[75] Crystal-induced arthritis Pseudogout[76]

composed of synovial fluid proteoglycans. Changes in this proteoglycan milieu, such as can occur with dilution, also will be noted and described.

It is important to remember that synovial fluid evaluation cannot be performed in isolation from other diagnostic tests. For example, a presumptive diagnosis of systemic lupus erythematosus requires more than cytologic observation of lupus erythematosus cells and ragocytes. Clinical signs, antinuclear antibody titers, and response to treatment also must be taken into account.[33] In addition, if rickettsial infection is suspected, it is recommended to perform both acute and convalescent serologic titers and polymerase chain reaction tests, as all tests can produce false negatives depending on the specific etiologic agent and stage of infection. Rarely, morulae can be observed in synovial fluid samples but specific identification of the rickettsial agent cannot be confirmed on cytology alone.[34–36] **Table 3** provides a summary of various arthropathies encountered in veterinary medicine.

REFERENCES

1. Braun JP, Bourges-Abella N, Geffre A, et al. The preanalytic phase in veterinary clinical pathology. Vet Clin Pathol 2015;44(1):8–25.

2. Gunn-Christie RG, Flatland B, Friedricks KR, et al. ASVCP quality assurance guidelines: control of preanalytical, analytical, and postanalytical factors for urinalysis, cytology, and clinical chemistry in veterinary laboratories. Vet Clin Pathol 2012;41(1):18–26.

3. Tomlinson L, Boone LI, Ramaiah L, et al. Best practices for veterinary toxicologic clinical pathology, with emphasis on the pharmaceutical and biotechnology industries. Vet Clin Pathol 2013;42(3):252–69.

4. Johnston SA. Osteoarthritis: joint anatomy, physiology, and pathobiology. Vet Clin North Am Small Anim Pract 1997;27:699–734.

5. Boon GD. Synovial fluid analysis: a guide for small-animal practitioners. Vet Med 1997;92:443–51.

6. Dearmin MG, Trumble TN, García A, et al. Chondroprotective effects of zoledronic acid on articular cartilage in dogs with experimentally induced osteoarthritis. Am J Vet Res 2014;75(4):329–37.

7. Fujita Y, Hara Y, Nezu Y, et al. Direct and indirect markers of cartilage metabolism in synovial fluid obtained from dogs with hip dysplasia and correlation with clinical and radiographic variables. Am J Vet Res 2005;66(12):2028–33.

8. Punzi L, Oliviero F. Arthrocentesis and synovial fluid analysis in clinical practice: value of sonography in difficult cases. Ann N Y Acad Sci 2009;1154:152–8.

9. Mach AJ, Adeyiga OB, Di Carlo D. Microfluidic sample preparation for diagnostic cytopathology. Lab Chip 2013;13(6):1011–26.

10. Jacques D, Cauzinille L, Bouvy B, et al. A retrospective study of 40 dogs with polyarthritis. Vet Surg 2002;31:428–34.

11. Pacchiana PD, Gilley RS, Wallace LJ, et al. Absolute and relative cell counts for synovial fluid from clinically normal shoulder and stifle joints in cats. J Am Vet Med Assoc 2004;225(12):1866–70.

12. Ogston AG, Sherman TF. Degradation of the hyaluronic acid complex of synovial fluid by proteolytic enzymes and by ethylenediaminetetra-acetic acid. Biochem J 1959;72:301–5.

13. Montgomery RD, Long IR, Milton JL, et al. Comparison of aerobic culturette, synovial membrane biopsy, and blood culture medium in detection of canine bacterial arthritis. Vet Surg 1989;18(4):300–3.

14. Berg RIM, Sykes JE, Kass PH, et al. Effect of repeated arthrocentesis on cytologic analysis of synovial fluid in dogs. J Vet Intern Med 2009;23:814–7.
15. Pedersen NC. Synovial fluid collection and analysis. Vet Clin North Am Small Anim Pract 1978;8(3):495–9.
16. MacWilliams PS, Friedrichs KR. Laboratory evaluation and interpretation of synovial fluid. Vet Clin North Am Small Anim Pract 2003;33:153–78.
17. Hardy RM, Wallace LJ. Arthrocentesis and synovial membrane biopsy. Vet Clin North Am Small Anim Pract 1974;4(2):449–62.
18. Sawyer DC. Synovial fluid analysis of canine joints. J Am Vet Med Assoc 1963; 143(6):609–12.
19. Fernandez FR, Grindem CB, Lipowitz AJ, et al. Synovial fluid analysis: preparation of smears for cytologic examination of canine synovial fluid. J Am Anim Hosp Assoc 1983;19:727–34.
20. Gibson NR, Carmichael S, Li A, et al. Value of direct smears of synovial fluid in the diagnosis of canine joint disease. Vet Rec 1999;144:463–5.
21. Ireifej SJ, Czaya CA, Flanders JA, et al. What is your diagnosis? Large juxta-articular soft tissue mass. J Am Vet Med Assoc 2007;230(9):1305–6.
22. Dougherty SA, Center SA, Shaw EE, et al. Juvenile-onset polyarthritis syndrome in akitas. J Am Vet Med Assoc 1991;198:849–56.
23. Schultz RM, Puchalski SM, Kent M, et al. Skeletal lesions of histiocytic sarcoma in nineteen dogs. Vet Radiol Ultrasound 2007;48(6):539–43.
24. Clements DN, Owen MR, Mosley JR, et al. Retrospective study of bacterial infective arthritis in 31 dogs. J Small Anim Pract 2005;46:171–6.
25. Brisson BA, Bersenas S, Etue SM. Ultrasonographic diagnosis of septic arthritis secondary to porcupine quill migration in a dog. J Am Vet Med Assoc 2004; 224(9):1467–70, 1453–4.
26. Marchevsky AM, Read RA. Bacterial septic arthritis in 19 dogs. Aust Vet J 1999; 77:233–7.
27. Rondeau MP, Walton RM, Bissett S, et al. Suppurative, nonseptic polyarthropathy in dogs. J Vet Intern Med 2005;19:654–62.
28. Barry SL, Lafuente MP, Martinez SA. Arthropathy caused by a lead bullet in a dog. J Am Vet Med Assoc 2008;232(6):886–8.
29. Ellison RS. The cytologic examination of synovial fluid. Semin Vet Med Surg 1988; 3(2):133–9.
30. Mills PC, Magnusson BM, Cross SE. Penetration of a topically applied nonsteroidal anti-inflammatory drug into local tissues and synovial fluid of dogs. Am J Vet Res 2005;66(7):1128–32.
31. Oke SL. Indications and contraindications for the use of orally administered joint health products in dogs and cats. J Am Vet Med Assoc 2009;234(11):1393–7.
32. Jones STM, Denton J, Holt PJL, et al. Refrigeration preserves synovial fluid cytology. Ann Rheum Dis 1993;52:384.
33. Melendez-Lazo A, Fernandez M, Solano-Gallego L, et al. What is your diagnosis? Synovial fluid from a dog. Vet Clin Pathol 2015;44(2):329–30.
34. Allison RW, Little SE. Diagnosis of rickettsial diseases in dogs and cats. Vet Clin Pathol 2013;42(2):127–44.
35. Gieg J, Rikihisa Y, Wellman M. Diagnosis of *Ehrlichia ewingii* infection by PCR in a puppy from Ohio. Vet Clin Pathol 2009;38(3):406–10.
36. Goodman RA, Hawkins EC, Olby NJ, et al. Molecular identification of *Ehrlichia ewingii* infection in dogs: 15 cases (1997-2001). J Am Vet Med Assoc 2003; 222(8):1102–7.

37. Atilola MAO, Lumsden JH, Rooke F. A comparison of manual and electronic counting for total nucleated cell counts on synovial fluid from canine stifle joints. Can J Vet Res 1986;50:282–4.
38. Barger AM. Musculoskeletal system. In: Raskin RE, Meyer DJ, editors. Canine and feline cytology: a color atlas and interpretation guide. 3rd edition. St Louis (MO): Elsevier; 2016. p. 353–68.
39. Carro T, Pedersen NC, Beaman BL, et al. Subcutaneous abscesses and arthritis caused by a probable bacterial L-form in cats. J Am Vet Med Assoc 1989; 194(11):1583–8.
40. Huss B, Collier L, Collins B, et al. Polyarthropathy and chorioretinitis with retinal detachment in a dog with systemic histoplasmosis. J Am Anim Hosp Assoc 1994;30:217–24.
41. Oxenford C, Middleton D. Osteomyelitis and arthritis associated with *Aspergillus fumigatus* in a dog. Aust Vet J 1986;63:59–61.
42. Johnson LR, Herrgesell EJ, Davidson AP, et al. Clinical, clinicopathologic, and radiographic findings in dogs with coccidioidomycosis: 24 cases (1995-2000). J Am Vet Med Assoc 2003;222(4):461–6.
43. Saito M, Sharp NJH, Munana K, et al. CT findings of intracranial blastomycosis in a dog. Vet Radiol Ultrasound 2002;43(1):16–21.
44. Headley SA, Mota FCD, Lindsay S, et al. *Cryptococcus neoformans* var. *grubii*-induced arthritis with encephalitic dissemination in a dog and review of published literature. Mycopathologia 2016;181:1–7.
45. Kornblatt AN, Urband PH, Steere AC. Arthritis caused by *Borrelia burgdorferi* in dogs. J Am Vet Med Assoc 1985;186(9):960–4.
46. Liehmann L, Degasperi B, Spergser J, et al. Mycoplasma felis arthritis in two cats. J Small Anim Pract 2006;47(8):476–9.
47. Barton MD, Ireland L, Kirschner JL, et al. Isolation of *Mycoplasma spumans* from polyarthritis in a greyhound. Aust Vet J 1985;62(6):206–7.
48. Santos M, Marcos R, Assunção M, et al. Polyarthritis associated with visceral leishmaniasis in a juvenile dog. Vet Parasitol 2006;141:340–4.
49. Cannon AB, Luff JA, Brault AC, et al. Acute encephalitis, polyarthritis, and myocarditis associated with West Nile virus infection in a dog. J Vet Intern Med 2006;20:1219–23.
50. Dawson S, Bennett D, Carter SD, et al. Acute arthritis of cats associated with feline calicivirus infection. Res Vet Sci 1994;56(2):133–43.
51. Levy J, Marsh A. Isolation of calicivirus from the joint of a kitten with arthritis. J Am Vet Med Assoc 1992;201:753–5.
52. Pedersen NC. A review of feline infectious peritonitis virus infection: 1963-2008. J Feline Med Surg 2009;11:225–58.
53. May C, Carter SD, Bell SC, et al. Immune responses to canine distemper virus in joint diseases of dogs. Rheumatology 1994;33(1):27–31.
54. Bennett D. Immune-based erosive inflammatory joint disease of the dog: canine rheumatoid arthritis. J Small Anim Pract 1987;28(9):799–819.
55. Woodard JC, Riser WH, Bloomberg MS, et al. Erosive polyarthritis in two greyhounds. J Am Vet Med Assoc 1991;198:873–6.
56. May C, Hammil J, Bennett D. Chinese shar pei fever syndrome: a preliminary report. Vet Rec 1992;131:586–7.
57. Oohashi E, Yamada K, Oohashi M, et al. Chronic progressive polyarthritis in a female cat. J Vet Med Sci 2010;72(4):511–4.
58. Pedersen N, Pool R, O'Brien T. Feline chronic progressive polyarthritis. Am J Vet Res 1980;41(4):522–35.

59. Silverstein DC, Almy FS, Zinkl JG, et al. Idiopathic localized eosinophilic synovitis in a cat. Vet Clin Pathol 2000;29(3):90–2.
60. Trepanier LA. Idiosyncratic toxicity associated with potentiated sulfonamides in the dog. J Vet Pharmacol Ther 2004;27:129–38.
61. Erne JB, Goring RL, Kennedy FA, et al. Prevalence of lymphoplasmacytic synovitis in dogs with naturally occurring cranial cruciate ligament rupture. J Am Vet Med Assoc 2009;235(4):386–90.
62. Kohn B, Garner M, Lübke S, et al. Polyarthritis following vaccination in four dogs. Vet Comp Orthop Traumatol 2003;16(1):6–10.
63. Bennett D, Kelly DF. Immune-based non-erosive inflammatory joint disease of the dog. 2. Polyarthritis/polymyositis syndrome. J Small Anim Pract 1987;28(10): 891–908.
64. Pereira PD, Santos M, Montenegro L, et al. A femorotibial joint swelling with popliteal lymph node enlargement in a rottweiler. Vet Clin Pathol 2006;35(3):335–8.
65. Moore PF. A review of histiocytic diseases of dogs and cats. Vet Pathol 2014; 51(1):167–84.
66. Pinard J, Wagg CR, Girard C, et al. Histiocytic sarcoma in the tarsus of a cat. Vet Pathol 2006;43(6):1014–7.
67. Craig LE, Julian ME, Ferracone JD. The diagnosis and prognosis of synovial tumors in dogs: 35 cases. Vet Pathol 2002;39(1):66–73.
68. Lowseth LA, Herbert RA, Muggenburg BA, et al. What is your diagnosis? Vet Clin Pathol 1989;18(3):57, 73–4.
69. Campbell MW, Koehler JW, Weiss RC, et al. Cytologic findings from a benign giant cell tumor of the tendon sheath in a dog. Vet Clin Pathol 2014;43(2):270–5.
70. Lahmers SM, Mealey KL, Martinez SA, et al. Synovial T-cell lymphoma of the stifle in a dog. J Am Anim Hosp Assoc 2002;38(2):165–8.
71. Thamm DH, Mauldin EA, Edinger DT, et al. Primary osteosarcoma of the synovium in a dog. J Am Anim Hosp Assoc 2000;36:326–31.
72. Miller MA, Pool RR, Coolman BR. Synovial hemangioma in the stifle joint of a dog. Vet Pathol 2007;44(2):240–3.
73. Colledge SL, Raskin RE, Messick JB, et al. Multiple joint metastasis of a transitional cell carcinoma in a dog. Vet Clin Pathol 2013;42(2):216–20.
74. Lowseth LA, Gillet NA, Muggenburg BA, et al. What is your diagnosis? Vet Clin Pathol 1989;18(4):88–9, 101–2.
75. Meinkoth JH, Rochat MC, Cowell RL. Metastatic carcinoma presenting as hindlimb lameness: diagnosis by synovial fluid cytology. J Am Anim Hosp Assoc 1997;33(4):325–8.
76. De Haan JJ, Andreasen CB. Calcium crystal-associated arthropathy (pseudogout) in a dog. J Am Vet Med Assoc 1992;200(7):943–6.

Analysis of Canine Peritoneal Fluid Analysis

Andrea A. Bohn, DVM, PhD

KEYWORDS

- Canine peritoneal fluid analysis • Effusion criteria • Transudate • Exudate

KEY POINTS

- The proposed classification scheme for canine peritoneal fluid analysis appears more effective than more complicated schemes.
- Low-protein transudates were most often caused by severe liver disease or protein-losing enteropathy.
- High-protein transudates were most often caused by heart failure and neoplasia.
- Exudates were most often caused by septic abdomen and neoplasia.
- Neoplasia can result in effusions in all classifications, as can uroabdomen; hemorrhagic and chylous effusions often are classified as exudates, but can be transudates as well.

PURPOSE

There is occasional criticism of the traditional classification of effusions and it is not clear how the published recommendations were established. This retrospective review of cases was performed to see how well a large number of canine peritoneal fluid analyses fit into previously published guidelines and to determine if there may be a simpler, more effective way to use fluid analysis in helping develop a differential list and diagnostic plan of action for dogs with peritoneal effusion.

BACKGROUND

Normal body cavity fluid is of low cell and protein concentrations (<3000 cells/μL and <2.5 g/dL, respectively) and is present in very small amounts.[1] When the amount of body cavity fluid is increased, it is called an effusion. An effusion occurs either because of increased fluid entering the cavity or decreased removal. The type of fluid varies depending on the underlying cause. It may have characteristics very similar to the normally present fluid, or it may have increased cellularity, increased protein,

The author has nothing to disclose.
Department of Microbiology, Immunology, and Pathology, College of Veterinary Medicine and Biomedical Sciences, Colorado State University, 1619 Campus Delivery, Fort Collins, CO 80523, USA
E-mail address: andrea.bohn@colostate.edu

Vet Clin Small Anim 47 (2017) 123–133
http://dx.doi.org/10.1016/j.cvsm.2016.07.008
0195-5616/17/© 2016 Elsevier Inc. All rights reserved.
vetsmall.theclinics.com

and/or presence of atypical cells or other substances. A definitive diagnosis is often not possible from fluid characteristics alone, but knowing the type of effusion can help prioritize differentials and direct additional diagnostics.

The small amount of normal body cavity fluid comes from submesothelial capillaries. There is normally a free exchange of water, electrolytes, and small molecules that occurs between the intravascular and extravascular spaces, the rate of which is largely controlled by hydrostatic and oncotic pressures within the capillaries. There is normally a net filtration from the capillaries, the excess of which is picked up by lymphatics. The permeability of mesothelium is similar to that of capillaries; therefore, after passing out of capillaries, fluid that is not reabsorbed can pass freely through submesothelial interstitium into peritoneal and pleural spaces. The permeability of capillary endothelium and mesothelium to proteins and cells is normally low. The submesothelial lymphatic system includes direct openings to the body cavities (stomas), located between mesothelial cells, which are important in reabsorption of fluid, cells, proteins, and particles.[2,3]

An effusion, then, can form due to changes in hydrostatic forces within the arteriolar or venous ends of capillaries, imbalance of oncotic pressures between capillaries and interstitium, increased vascular or mesothelial permeability, or decreased lymphatic reabsorption of the fluid. Addition of fluid from other sources, such as leakage from the blood or lymphatic vasculature, urinary bladder, or biliary tract, can also result in an effusion. Of course, multiple factors may be present at the same time.

Transudates are often the result of changes in oncotic or hydrostatic pressure or decreased reabsorption; they have low total nucleated cell concentrations (TNCC) with variable total protein concentrations ([TP]) depending on cause and whether they arise before or after liver sinusoids. Oncotic pressure is largely dependent on plasma albumin concentration. Changes in capillary or lymphatic hydrostatic pressure can be systemic but are often more localized due to compression of vasculature from mass lesions or organ displacement, torsion, or distension, or due to intravascular blockage from thrombi or neoplasia. Exudates are most often associated with increased vascular permeability due to inflammation, resulting in high TNCC and [TP]. There are other fluids with increased cellularity that may not be exudates, technically, but, based on cell counts, we include them in the exudative category for convenience; these include neoplastic, lymphatic, and hemorrhagic effusions. Effusions caused by leakage of fluid from vessels or organs can result in variable fluid composition depending on quantity, chronicity, and other factors and therefore may fall into either the transudate or exudate category.

Effusions have traditionally been characterized based on TNCC and [TP], with cell types and a few other characteristics taken into account. In veterinary medicine, transudates are typically subcategorized as either a pure transudate or modified transudate. In small animals, the parameters recommended for pure transudates range from less than 1000 to 1500 cells/μL with less than 2.5 g/dL protein and those for modified transudates are a [TP] greater than 2.5 g/dL and TNCC either less than 5000 or from 1000 to 7000/μL.[4–6] Exudates are described as [TP] greater than 2.0, 2.5, or 3.0 g/dL and the TNCC as greater than 3000, 5000, or 7000/μL, depending on source.[4–8] In one source, modified transudates represent any fluid that does not fit their parameters for either a transudate (TNCC <3000/μL and [TP] <2.5 g/dL) or exudate (TNCC >3000/μL and [TP] >2.5 g/dL).[7] Another source uses a [TP] of 2.0 mg/dL to differentiate between low-protein and high-protein transudates.[8] Given the variability in pathologic processes, is it possible that having multiple cutoffs and too many restrictions has complicated the process of fluid analysis and resulted in more confusion than necessary in their classification; is there an easier way?

THE STUDY

This retrospective study was performed by searching for all canine peritoneal fluid analyses run on in-hospital patients from July 1, 2014, to July 1, 2015. Only the first sample from each animal was used if multiple samples were collected. All samples included were from different dogs except one who returned weeks after the first admission with a different disease process. Data extracted from the medical record and entered into an Excel spreadsheet included the description of fluid quantity based on focused assessment with sonography in trauma (FAST) scan, full abdominal ultrasound, or surgery report, peritoneal fluid analysis results (color and clarity of fluid and supernatant, TNCC, [TP] by refractometer, red blood cell concentration [RBC], nucleated cell differential, comments on cell populations or other findings, and pathologist interpretation), serum albumin, and diagnosis. All samples were then reclassified as transudate, modified transudate and exudate using [TP] less than 2.5 g/dL and TNCC less than 1000/µL, [TP] 2.5 g/dL or greater and TNCC less than 5000/µL, and [TP] greater than 3.0 g/dL and TNCC greater than or equal to 5000/µL, respectively.[6] Samples that did not fit these criteria were categorized separately.

Assessing Cutoff Criteria

Using the previously mentioned criteria,[6] there were 25 transudates, 30 modified transudates, and 33 exudates. For fluids that did not fall within the criteria, there were 9 cases with [TP] less than 2.5 g/dL and TNCC greater than 1000/µL (5 of these with >5000 cells/µL) and 8 cases with [TP] of 2.5 to 3.0 g/dL and TNCC greater than 5000/µL.

Based on initial observations, there did not appear to be any advantage in using cellularity (<1000 or 1500 vs 1000–5000 cells/µL) to differentiate between the 2 different types of transudates or their underlying disease processes. To determine a more precise cutoff between transudates and exudates, cases that had TNCC between the lower and upper published limits for categorization as an exudate (3000–7000/µL) were evaluated and it appeared that 3000 may be a better cutoff value. Of the 10 cases that had cell counts in that range, 6 had an inflammatory component to their cause. There were also 2 cases of neoplasia, which can fall into any classification, and 1 case each of lymphangiectasia and idiopathic effusion.

Reclassification

Cases were subsequently recategorized by first classifying the fluid as a transudate (TNCC <3000/µL) or exudate (TNCC ≥3000/µL) and then splitting the transudates into low-protein or high-protein categories (<2.5 and ≥2.5 g/dL, respectively).

Results of peritoneal fluid analyses and disease processes were evaluated and compared with previous recommended fluid analysis guidelines. Data were sorted in multiple ways to look for obvious trends. As an observational study, no statistics were performed.

RESULTS

There were 107 samples from 106 dogs. Most fluids were similarly categorized regardless of which method of classification was used; however, there was less ambiguity in classifying a low number of cases when using the TNCC of 3000/µL and [TP] of

2.5 g/dL cutoff values; this TNCC also better identified inflammatory processes without causing any detrimental misclassifications. Several disease processes were nicely split out when using a TNCC of 3000/μL and [TP] of 2.5 g/dL for the classification of canine peritoneal effusions, as can be seen in **Table 1**.

Severe liver disease and protein-losing enteropathy were the most common causes of low-protein transudates. Heart failure was the most common cause of high-protein transudates. Septic abdomen was the most common cause of exudates. Neoplasia was the most common cause of effusion overall, with cases falling within all effusion classifications. The most common organs implicated in peritoneal effusions are the gastrointestinal (GI) tract, liver, and heart. Of course, prevalence of the different causes of effusion will likely vary between different types of practices and geographic locations. For example, none of the dogs in this study had heartworm disease, which is a common cause of heart failure with secondary effusion in the southeast United States. Fortunately, although diagnostic efforts are initially typically focused on ruling in or out the more common causes, less common causes can be looked for concurrently.

Table 1
Classification of 107 canine peritoneal fluids based on cutoffs of 3000/μL TNCC and 2.5 g/dL [TP], grouped according to cause

Diagnosis	Low-Protein Transudate, TNCC <3000/μL, [TP] <2.5 mg/dL	High-Protein Transudate, TNCC <3000/μL, [TP] ≥2.5 mg/dL	Exudate, TNCC ≥3000/μL
Liver failure/portal hypertension	8	—	—
Protein-losing enteropathy	7	—	—
Vasculitis	1[a]	—	—
Splenic vein thrombosis	1	1	—
Enteritis	4[a]	2[a,b]	—
Heart failure	—	10[a]	—
GI displacement	—	2	—
GI foreign body	—	2	1
Uroabdomen	1	1	2
Neoplasia	3	9	14[a,b]
Septic abdomen	—	—	17[a]
Postoperative (2 with pancreatitis)	—	—	7[a]
Pancreatitis	—	—	4[a,b]
Bile peritonitis	—	—	1
Biliary obstruction/cholecystitis	—	—	1
Splenic hematoma with necrosis	—	—	1
Lymphangiectasia	—	—	1
Undetermined	2	2	2

Abbreviations: GI, gastrointestinal; RBC, red blood cell; TNCC, total nucleated cell concentration; [TP], total protein concentration.
[a] Categories having at least one fluid containing evidence of previous hemorrhage with RBC/μL <500,000.
[b] Categories that contained at least 1 fluid described as hemorrhagic (RBC/μL >500,000).

Observations

Protein

Most exudates had increased protein, however 6 samples had a [TP] lower than 2.5 g/dL. Two of these were cases of uroabdomen, 2 had a septic abdomen, and 2 samples were collected postoperatively (1 of these cases also may have had pancreatitis and/or liver failure), therefore low-protein concentration obviously does not rule out a primary inflammatory process.

Using a 2.0 versus 2.5 g/dL [TP] cutoff did not appear discriminating between high and low transudate causes. For example, using 2.0 g/dL [TP] as a cutoff, 2 enteritis and 2 neoplasia samples moved to the high-protein category, but there were still effusions caused by enteritis and neoplasia that remained classified as low-protein transudates. Therefore, a cutoff of 2.5 g/dL was used. Because 2.5 g/dL is the upper limit for [TP] in normal peritoneal fluid, this scheme helps to simplify classification of fluids in small animals.

It has been stated that most mammals with a protein-poor transudate will have a serum albumin less than 1.5 g/dL.[8] Only 1 dog in this case study had a fluid protein of 1.4 g/dL. All other dogs had serum albumin of 1.5 g/dL or higher. Several dogs with protein-losing enteropathy (PLE) and low-protein transudates had serum albumin of 1.5 to 1.8 g/dL. There were also several cases in which fluid protein was less than 1.0 g/dL and serum albumin was 1.9 to 2.5 g/dL. It is likely that in many of these cases a combination of oncotic and hydrostatic pressure changes is contributing to the effusion; several had severe chronic liver disease. Oncotic pressure differences may not be high enough to result in effusion, despite marked hypoalbuminemia if interstitial protein content is also low. Rapid drops in serum albumin concentration may more likely lead to transudation, which may occur after fluid therapy.

Neutrophils

It is often suggested that transudates should have less than 50% neutrophils and 1 source states that neutrophils are rarely greater than 30% in modified transudates.[6] This appears to be inaccurate and the percent neutrophils does not appear to contribute much to the evaluation of transudates. In this study, only 8 of 28 low-protein and 1 of 27 high-protein transudates had neutrophils less than 30%; more than half of all transudates had neutrophils greater than 50% with a maximum of 88% (excluding a case of uroabdomen and a case of necrotic hepatocellular carcinoma, each at 92%). Although there may be mild inflammatory processes occurring, recognition of such does not help differentiate between the potential underlying primary processes creating the transudate. Calling these effusions inflammatory is more likely to create confusion than help determine the underlying pathogenesis.

Eosinophils

In this set of cases, the presence of eosinophils was most often associated with lesions of the digestive system, including 4 cases of PLE. Hemorrhagic effusions were also frequently associated with low numbers of eosinophils. Effusions due to heart failure frequently contained eosinophils and had the highest percent at 26%. All other cases had less than 10% eosinophils except for a case of eosinophilic enteritis at 10%. Although not detected in this study, eosinophilic effusions also can be associated with allergic hypersensitivity conditions, parasitic disease, and neoplasms, including lymphoma and mast cell neoplasia.[9]

Lymphocytes
There were only 7 cases that had lymphocytes 30% or higher and only 1 of these fell into the exudate category, a case of lymphangiectasia with a fluid TNCC of 3200/µL. Two of the 6 transudates with lymphocytes 30% or higher had atypical large lymphocytes present, consistent with the diagnosis of intestinal and hepatosplenic lymphoma. Another case was diagnosed with lymphoma causing PLE, but the small lymphocytes seen in the peritoneal fluid were likely due to concurrent lymphangiectasia rather than representing a neoplastic cell population. The remaining cases with lymphocytes greater than or equal to 30% were diagnosed with enteritis. Of the 8 cases that had lymphocytes between 20% and 30%, one had lymphoblasts in the fluid despite having only 100 cells/µL. The remaining cases had a variety of diagnoses that led to effusions.

Fluid quantity
Because ultrasonography is used so much more often now than when fluid analysis parameters were initially published, and cases with mild effusion would likely have been missed in the past, the amount of fluid detected (mild, moderate, or marked, as subjectively described in the medical record) was compared with fluid classifications and disease processes. The most common causes of marked fluid accumulation were liver failure/portal hypertension, severe heart disease, and neoplasia. There were also some cases of septic abdomen and a case of uroabdomen with marked fluid accumulation. Most dogs with PLE had moderate fluid accumulation. Otherwise, most causes of effusion were pretty evenly split between mild and moderate quantities. A handful of cases did not have an effusion at presentation, but developed mild effusion after intravenous fluid administration; most of these cases were exudates associated with pancreatitis or septic abdomen and a few dogs became moderately hypoalbuminemic after fluid therapy.

Fluid color
Although useful, color descriptions did not appear to have strong associations with any particular disease process in this study. In the case of bile peritonitis, the fluid was described as orange and opaque with an orange and hazy supernatant, but other, non–bile-related cases were described similarly. White and opaque fluids are classic for chylous effusions, but no samples fit this description in this case study, supporting the belief that peritoneal chylous effusions are uncommon.

Bicavitary effusions
Besides the 5 cases of pericardial effusion, other causes of bicavitary effusion included 2 cases of heart failure, 3 cases of neoplasia, 1 case of vasculitis, and 1 case of lymphangiectasia. There was also 1 case of idiopathic bicavitary effusion that resolved.

Various Causes of Effusion

Hemorrhage
Of the hemorrhagic effusions in this study (defined as >500,000 RBC/µL), 6 of 7 fell within the exudate category; 5 had neoplasia and 1 had pancreatitis. The fluids were relatively easily identified as hemorrhagic and some had an obvious inflammatory component as well. The hemorrhagic sample with low TNCC and [TP] came from a dog with severe gastroenteritis and hemorrhagic diarrhea. Fluids with [RBC] greater than 150,000/µL were consistently associated with previous hemorrhage rather than

blood contamination and those with [RBC] greater than 200,000/µL were associated with neoplasia, pancreatitis, or septic abdomen. There were other fluids with lower numbers of erythrocytes (0–70,000/µL) but with evidence of previous hemorrhage (macrophages containing erythrocytes and/or hemosiderin). These included 5 cases of heart failure/pericardial effusion, 3 cases of neoplasia, 1 case of hemorrhagic gastro-enteritis, 1 septic abdomen, and 1 effusion caused by vasculitis. Hemorrhagic effusions may occur from trauma or torsion causing rupture of a vessel or organ as well as the diseases listed here. Bleeding diatheses can also lead to hemorrhagic effusions.

Lymph
Chylous effusions are not common for canine abdominal fluids. When lymph fluid contains chyle (largely composed of chylomicrons from the small intestinal lacteals after fat digestion), it often has a characteristic milky appearance. Chylous effusions can also appear more serous. If wanting to confirm the fluid is chylous, the cholesterol-triglyceride ratio (<1) or, even better, just the triglyceride concentration (>100 mg/dL) of the fluid can be measured.[5–8] There are also lymphatic effusions that are not chylous: if the animal has not recently ingested a fatty meal or if the lymphatics affected are not draining the intestinal tract. The same underlying disease processes can cause both and, in fact, are the same processes that can lead to transfusions in general. Increased hydrostatic pressure within or increased permeability of lymphatic vessels can lead to lymphatic leakage from vessels, as well as can physical damage to the vessels.

Chylous/lymphatic effusions may fall into either the transudate or exudate categories based on cell counts, although differentials are typically more in line with transudates. Increased proportions of lymphocytes are expected, although they may not be the predominant cell. In this case study, no obvious chylous effusions were detected, but lymphangiectasia was diagnosed in one and expected in at least one other case; these cases had 55% lymphocytes of a 3200/µL TNCC and 37% of a 200/µL TNCC, respectively. It would not be surprising to occasionally have a small contribution of lymph in effusions, given the close association of blood and lymph vessels and similar underlying mechanisms leading to increased fluid.

It is important to assess cell morphology in all fluid samples. There were 3 samples in this study that, despite having low TNCC, intermediate to large, immature lymphocytes were observed, indicative of lymphoma. Interestingly, all cases of lymphoma in this study were transudates.

Urine
Uroabdomen can have variable peritoneal fluid characteristics and be associated with either high or low-protein transudates or exudates as seen in this group of cases. Fluid characteristics are likely influenced by how much urine has leaked, for how long, and its cause. The typical way to confirm suspected uroabdomen is to collect time-matched blood and urine samples for creatinine measurements. The creatinine concentration in urine should be at least 2 times that of serum or plasma. Additionally, urine [K+]–serum [K+] ratio should be greater than 1.4.[10] Of the 4 uroabdomen cases in this study, the amount of fluid ranged from mild to marked, TNCC ranged from 50/µL to 6000/µL, [TP] from 0.3 to 2.6 g/dL, and percent neutrophils from 68% to 93%.

Neoplasia
Effusions caused by neoplasia can be high-protein or low-protein transudates or exudates because the potential effusive mechanisms are varied, although the vast majority have increased protein. Although neoplastic cells may be present in the effusion, in most cases the effusion is caused by compromise to blood and lymphatic

---

Box 1
Initial analysis of canine peritoneal fluid

1. Evaluate the cell count:
   a. If ≥3000/μL, see **Box 2**
   b. If <3000/μL, measure [TP]
      i. If [TP] <2.5 g/dL, see **Box 3**
      ii. If [TP] ≥2.5 g/dL, see **Box 4**

Tip: If samples are submitted to an outside laboratory, send a few freshly made slides with the fluid sample to minimize confusion from in vitro artifact.

---

vasculature resulting in a transudate or hemorrhagic effusion. Effusions may be inflammatory, especially if there is inflammation or necrosis in the tumor. In this case study, and as previously described, carcinoma was the most common diagnosis when neoplastic cells were present in the effusion.

Gastrointestinal
Compromise to the bowel often results in a transudate, likely due to vascular effects. But if compromise is severe, resulting in tissue injury or necrosis, an exudate is likely to form.

Septic inflammation
The highest number of septic peritonitis cases was associated with GI perforation after nonsteroidal anti-inflammatory drug therapy or was seen postoperatively after various surgical procedures. A few cases were also caused by ruptured tumors of the gut and liver or GI foreign bodies. The amount of effusion ranged from mild to marked. TNCC

Box 2
Working up an exudate (TNCC ≥3000/μL)

1. Microscopic examination:
   a. Predominantly neutrophils:
      i. Look for microorganisms, foreign material
      ii. Consider whether surgery or diagnostic radiology imaging is indicated (see **Box 5**)
      iii. Consider whether additional testing for bile peritonitis, uroabdomen, pancreatitis, or sepsis is indicated (see **Box 6**)
   b. Neoplastic cells are present:
      i. Diagnostic radiology imaging for localizing the neoplasm; aspirate for cytology if appropriate or biopsy with histologic examination for confirmation of neoplasia and tissue of origin
   c. High number of red blood cells (RBCs) present (also evaluate RBC count/hematocrit):
      i. Rule out blood contamination (platelets present and no erythrophagocytosis or hemosiderin)
      ii. Evaluate for neoplasia, pancreatitis, and septic abdomen
      iii. If coagulopathy is a possible underlying cause, complete blood count/platelet count and coagulation panel are indicated
   d. High proportion of lymphocytes present:
      i. A lymphoproliferative disorder is present if lymphocytes are immature
      ii. If lymphocytes are small with mature chromatin, consider PARR (polymerase chain reaction for antigen receptor rearrangements) or flow cytometry to rule out a small cell lymphoproliferative disorder, especially if lymphocytes are greater than 10,000/μL
      iii. Probable lymphatic effusion
         1. Possible lymphangiectasia
         2. See **Box 4**
         3. If want to assess whether chylous, see **Box 6**

Box 3
Working up low-protein transudates: total nucleated cell concentrations ([TNCC] <3000/μL and total protein concentrations [TP] <2.5 g/dL)

1. Microscopic examination
   a. Neoplastic cells are present:
      i. Diagnostic radiology imaging for localizing the neoplasm; aspirate for cytology if appropriate or biopsy with histologic examination for confirmation of neoplasia and tissue of origin
   b. In absence of neoplasia, nucleated cell differential usually not discriminatory

2. Serum biochemistry analysis
   a. Serum albumin: if low, evaluate for protein-losing disease processes
      i. Gastrointestinal (GI) evaluation/testing
      ii. Urinalysis
   b. Liver enzymes and function tests

3. Diagnostic radiology imaging if no cause detected or if further evaluation of liver or GI desired (see **Box 5**)

Box 4
Working up high-protein transudates: TNCC <3000/μL and [TP] ≥2.5 g/dL

1. Microscopic examination
   a. Neoplastic cells are present:
      i. Diagnostic radiology imaging for localizing the neoplasm; aspirate for cytology if appropriate or biopsy with histologic examination for confirmation of neoplasia and tissue of origin
   b. In absence of neoplasia, nucleated cell differential usually not discriminatory

2. Rule out heart failure

3. Consider GI causes

4. Radiological imaging if no cause detected or if further evaluation of GI desired (see **Box 5**)

Box 5
Steps to take if no cause of effusion is obvious

1. Consider uroabdomen (see **Box 6**)

2. Ultrasonography ± radiography are useful tools in assessing abdominal structures. Depending on findings, additional diagnostics may be indicated.
   a. Neoplasia is a common cause of effusion and can arise in any tissue
      i. Aspiration or biopsy of mass lesions, as appropriate
   b. Assessment of spleen and hepatobiliary and genitourinary systems
   c. GI defects, distension, displacement, foreign bodies
   d. Pancreas; pancreatitis (see **Box 6**)
   e. Vascular thrombi

Box 6
Additional testing

If suspect:

1. Uroabdomen: Fluid [creatinine] >2× serum [creatinine]; fluid [K+] >1.4× serum [K+] are indicative[10]

2. Bile peritonitis: Fluid [bilirubin] > serum [bilirubin][6]; if bilirubin results are equivocal, measuring fluid versus serum [bile acids] may be useful[11]

3. Pancreatitis: Peritoneal fluid [cPLI] >500 μg/L, fluid [lipase] >500 U/L, or fluid [lipase] >2× serum [lipase] are supportive of pancreatitis[12,13]

4. Chylous effusion: fluid cholesterol-triglyceride ratio <1; fluid [triglyceride] >100 mg/dL are indicative[5–8]

5. Septic peritonitis: A blood-to-fluid glucose difference >20 mg/dL and blood-to-fluid lactate difference <2.0 mmol/L were highly sensitive and specific for septic peritonitis, which could be useful in suspected cases in which bacteria are not seen[14]

---

ranged from 8600 to 194,000/μL and [TP] from 0.1 to 4.6 g/dL. The proportion of neutrophils in these samples ranged from 77% to 100%.

DISCUSSION

Based on these 107 samples, there did not appear to be any benefit in having multiple cutoffs for TNCC or [TP] in the classification of canine peritoneal effusions and using a TNCC of 3000/μL appeared most appropriate for distinguishing transudates from exudates. There will likely be some fluids that will defy these numbers once more cases are assessed, but should be no worse, and likely slightly better, than using the current system. Further studies are needed to determine if these simplified cutoffs will work for thoracic cavity effusions and in cats as well.

The whole point of analyzing body cavity effusions is to help determine why the effusion occurred. Determining TNCC and [TP] is only the first step in fluid characterization and, although these values will lead to an initial classification that may cause one to begin conjuring a differential list, a final classification cannot occur without microscopic examination and, possibly, additional testing. To complicate matters, there are several processes that can result in more than 1 classification of effusion. Numerical data need to be interpreted in context with the types of cells present and what is occurring clinically. Microscopic findings, including cell distribution, atypical cells, degenerative changes of neutrophils, previous hemorrhage, infectious agents, or foreign material are imperative to interpretation and may outweigh numerical data in classifying and determining the cause of an effusion.

Recommendations

Recommended steps to take during and after evaluation of body cavity effusions are displayed in **Boxes 1–6**. Of course, patient signalment, clinical signs, physical examination findings, laboratory data, and history will greatly influence which steps are most appropriate.

REFERENCES

1. O'Brien PJ, Lumsden JH. The cytologic examination of body cavity fluids. Semin Vet Med Surg 1988;3:140–56.

2. Zocchi L. Physiology and pathophysiology of pleural fluid turnover. Eur Respir J 2002;20:1545–58.
3. Aguirre AR, Abensur H. Physiology of fluid and solute transport across the peritoneal membrane. J Bras Nefrol 2014;36:74–9.
4. Valenciano AC, Arndt TP, Rizzi TE. Effusions: abdominal, thoracic, and pericardial. In: Valenciano AC, Cowell RL, editors. Cowell and Tyler's diagnostic cytology and hematology of the dog and cat. 4th edition. St. Louis (MO): Mosby; 2014. p. 244–65.
5. Rakich PM, Latimer KS. Cytology. In: Latimer KS, editor. Duncan & Prasse's veterinary laboratory medicine: clinical pathology. 5th edition. Ames (IA): Wiley-Blackwell; 2011. p. 331–63.
6. Thompson CA, Rebar AH. Body cavity fluids. In: Raskin RE, Meyer DJ, editors. Canine and feline cytology: a color atlas and interpretation guide. 3rd edition. Philadelphia: WB Saunders; 2015. p. 191–219.
7. Baker R, Lumsden JH. Pleural and peritoneal fluids. In: Baker R, Lumsden JH, editors. Color atlas of cytology of the dog and cat. St. Louis (MO): Mosby; 2000. p. 159–65.
8. Stockam SL, Scott MA. Cavitary effusions. In: Stockham SL, Scott MA, editors. Fundamentals of veterinary clinical pathology. 2nd edition. Ames (IA): Blackwell Publishing; 2008. p. 831–68.
9. Fossum TW, Wellman M, Relford R, et al. Eosinophilic pleural or peritoneal effusions in dogs and cats: 14 cases (1986–1992). J Am Vet Med Assoc 1993;202: 1873–6.
10. Schmiedt C, Tobias KM, Otto CM. Evaluation of abdominal fluid: peripheral blood creatinine and potassium ratios for diagnosis of uroperitoneum in dogs. JVECC 2001;11:275–80.
11. Guess SC, Harkin KR, Biller DS. Anicteric gallbladder rupture in dogs: 5 cases (2007–2013). J Am Vet Med Assoc 2015;247:1412–4.
12. Chartier MA, Hill SL, Sunico S, et al. Pancreas-specific lipase concentrations and amylase and lipase activities in the peritoneal fluid of dogs with suspected pancreatitis. Vet J 2014;201:385–9.
13. Guija de Arespacochaga A, Hittmair KM, Schwendenwein I. Comparison of lipase activity in peritoneal fluid of dogs with different pathologies–a complementary diagnostic tool in acute pancreatitis? J Vet Med A Physiol Pathol Clin Med 2006;53:119–22.
14. Bonczynski JJ, Ludwig LL, Barton LJ, et al. Comparison of peritoneal fluid and peripheral blood pH, bicarbonate, glucose, and lactate concentration as a diagnostic tool for septic peritonitis in dogs and cats. Vet Surg 2003;32:161–6.

Urine Cytology
Collection, Film Preparation, and Evaluation

Linda M. Vap, DVM[a],*, Sarah B. Shropshire, DVM[b]

KEYWORDS

- Transitional cell carcinoma • Urine collection • Bacteriuria • Voided • Cystocentesis
- Culture

KEY POINTS

- Cytologic examination of the urine sediment in animals suspected of having urinary tract disease and/or lower urinary tract masses is one of the best means of distinguishing inflammation, infection, and neoplasia and it can help determine if a positive dipstick result for hemoglobin/blood is due to hemorrhage or blood contamination.
- The quality of the specimen collection and handling plays an important role in the quality of results, the validity of interpretations, and selection of appropriate course of action.
- The method of sample collection aids localization of pathology.
- Air dry, but do not heat fix, freeze, or expose films to formalin fumes, temperature extremes, or condensation.

INTRODUCTION

Urinalysis is an important part of the minimum database for routine health screens and is used as a means of monitoring response to treatment. Although a complete urinalysis provides a critical indication of renal function, acid-base homeostasis, and other body systems, the focus of this article is the cytologic examination of urine sediment for evidence of inflammation, infection, and/or neoplasia. It can also help determine if a positive dipstick result for hemoglobin/blood is due to hemorrhage or blood contamination. The specific method of sample collection can assist with localizing the source of pathology when interpreted with the cytologic findings. Images of urine sediment are included that illustrate common findings in these samples.

The authors have nothing to disclose.

[a] Department of Microbiology, Immunology, and Pathology, College of Veterinary Medicine and Biomedical Sciences, Colorado State University, 300 West Drake Road, Fort Collins, CO 80523, USA; [b] Department of Clinical Sciences, College of Veterinary Medicine and Biomedical Sciences, Colorado State University, 300 West Drake Road, Fort Collins, CO 80523, USA
* Corresponding author.
E-mail address: Linda.Vap@ColoState.EDU

LABORATORY MEDICINE ROLE

Urine cytology continues to comprise largely manual microscopic methods. Much can be done with a quality microscope in the hands of experienced personnel. Digital imagery can be submitted to a clinical pathologist for further evaluation. A few recent developments, such as rapid manual tests for determining the presence and Gram-staining characteristics of bacteria and presence of transitional cell carcinoma complement the manual techniques. A recently marketed automated sediment analyzer claims the ability to evaluate urine for blood and epithelial cells, bacteria, casts, and common crystals.

CLINICAL PRESENTATION

Indications for cytologic evaluation of urine and the lower urinary tract include routine screening as part of the minimum database or a pursuit for an explanation of polydipsia, polyuria, pollakiuria, pain, discolored urine, dysuria, anorexia, and/or vomiting. Mass lesions or other abnormalities discovered by palpation or imaging in the bladder or distal urinary tract are other reasons for cytologic evaluation of this region. The risks of obtaining a urine or tissue samples are generally considered minimal and are related to the method of collection as provided in the tables.

SPECIMEN PROCUREMENT/TRACKING

As with most laboratory procedures, the quality of the specimen collection and handling plays an important role in the quality of results, validity of interpretations and therapeutic selections.[1] Urine collection containers should be clean, sterile, and constructed of nonbreakable, leak-proof material, such as plastic cups with a screw top lid commercially sold for this purpose. Syringes are acceptable when the samples are collected by cystocentesis or catheterization; however, it must be insured that the needle is snugly capped or replaced with a clean syringe cap to avoid sample contamination. Owners should be warned against using food or other reused containers because these may not be sterile and detergents can interfere with biochemical results. If there is a potential for zoonotic infectious agents, medical professionals should collect the sample using biosafety precautions and insure the specimen is properly labeled as potentially biohazardous.

The source of formed elements observed in urine varies with the method of collection. Collection options, selection criteria, advantages, and disadvantages are provided in **Boxes 1–3**.[2]

Voided, or free catch, specimens may be obtained by holding the collection receptacle near the urethral opening during micturition. This may be easier said than done but is feasible in many veterinary patients. Using a receptacle other than a bulky urine specimen cup can address problems collecting samples. Examples include a flat rectangular clean plastic container (Tupperware, for example) or a clean ladle spoon (recommended). The urine is then poured into the sterile urine specimen cup as soon as possible. Collapsible sticks or poles that hold the receptacle of choice in place allow owners to adjust the length so that the dog can urinate multiple feet away (as normal on a leash) and they can still catch the urine. If urine is voided onto the floor, it can be aspirated using a sterile syringe and needle but such samples are prone to significant contamination. Manual bladder expression is not recommended because this can induce trauma/discomfort to the patient, force bacterial organisms into other urogenital areas, and result in hemorrhage that complicates interpretation of the urinalysis (**Box 1**).

Box 1
Voided/free catch (first stream, midstream, collected off floor)

For: urethral pathology (first stream), hematuria, routine screening

Localization: urogenital tract

Advantages: owner can obtain, minimally invasive. Minimize contamination (midstream). Litter options aid collection in cats. May be only means available (severe pollakiuria). Fresh cell morphology (random timing).

Disadvantages: external urethral (male), urogenital, fecal (female), and/or floor/table contamination; not recommended for culture. More challenging in female patients (low posturing), small or chondrodysplastic breeds, and cats unfamiliar with new litter substrate in home environment.

There are several ways to collect a cystocentesis sample, which include via ultrasound guidance, manual palpation with immobilization of the urinary bladder, or a blind technique. It is considered preferable to be able to visualize the urinary bladder via ultrasound or manually palpate it before attempting a cystocentesis because the blind technique can have serious complications (described later). For samples collected via ultrasound guidance, canine patients can be in left or right lateral recumbency, dorsal recumbency, or standing whereas feline patients can be in either left or right lateral recumbency or dorsal recumbency but this should not be attempted while standing in cats. The angle of the needle is typically directed at an oblique angle to the ultrasound probe and the needle entry into the urinary bladder is visualized. For cystocentesis samples collected via manual palpation, most dogs and cats are placed in left or right lateral recumbency simply because it is easier to immobilize the urinary bladder in this position. This technique can also be performed in standing or in dorsal recumbency if the patient is very well-mannered or is at an ideal body weight. The angle of the needle depends on the position of the patient and how the bladder is immobilized. For a thin cat in lateral recumbency, the needle is held at a 90° angle to the skin whereas in a dog in dorsal recumbency, the needle is often held at an oblique angle (directed caudally) to try to enter the urinary bladder lumen directly.[3] The blind cystocentesis technique is typically done in canine patients because the urinary bladder can be palpated readily in most cats or it is visualized via ultrasound. This technique can be done in dorsal recumbency or standing in dogs. In dorsal recumbency, there are 2 methods that can be used to successfully collect a sample. The first method involves pouring a small amount of alcohol on the caudal abdomen on midline and seeing where the alcohol pools. This can be where the urinary bladder is located but this is not always reliable because the bladder may be more cranially or caudally located in some patients or the urinary bladder is simply empty. The excess alcohol is dabbed away with cotton or gauze before insertion of the needle. The second method includes inserting the needle on midline halfway between the pelvic brim and umbilicus or on midline at the location where a theoretic line would be drawn between where the last 2 sets of nipples would cross. When using the blind technique in male patients, the prepuce is often moved to the side to gain access to midline. The angle of the needle can be at an oblique angle to the skin (the needle enters the bladder cranially and is directed toward the trigone) or is more often directed at a 90° angle to the skin. For dogs, the blind technique can be done in standing as well. This is done by palpating the caudal abdomen for a divot or indention along midline and this is where the needle is inserted at a 90° angle. This is the same location where alcohol often pools or is the halfway point between the umbilicus and pelvic brim. Regardless of the technique for cystocentesis, consistent negative pressure should be applied while collecting the urine but no suction should be present when removing the needle to decrease the chance of aspirating abdominal contents or fat, which could contaminate the sample.[4] If blood is seen in the hub of the needle, the needle should be immediately removed (with no suction) and the procedure should be repeated with a new sterile needle and syringe. Another consideration when collecting a sample via cystocentesis is whether to use alcohol or not to aseptically prepare the site. The general recommendation is to move excess hair out of the way with an alcohol swab but these samples are often collected without clipping or aseptically preparing the site because this can sometimes result in clipper burn or irritation to the skin and potentially compromise the site. Although this technique is an efficient way to collect urine, it is also important to consider whether it is appropriate to use in each individual patient (**Box 2**).

Urethral catheterization requires trained personnel knowledgeable in sterile techniques.

Catheterization of male dogs typically requires 2 people and is done with the patient in left or right lateral recumbency. One person wearing nonsterile gloves moves the prepuce back gently to expose the penis and then the penis is aseptically prepped with a gentle cleansing solution. The penis remains unsheathed while the other person atraumatically places a sterile urinary catheter. This catheter would have been previously measured for appropriate length and diameter for the patient. The person placing the urinary catheter wears sterile gloves and uses sterile lube along the length of the catheter to help with placement. Once the urinary catheter is estimated to be in the urinary bladder, urine either starts to leak from the catheter or a sterile syringe can be used to aspirate and obtain a sample. Once the sample is obtained, the urinary catheter is gently removed. In female patients, the vulva is clipped of excess hair and aseptically prepped with a dilute chlorhexidine solution or other gentle cleansing solution.[3] Placement can be performed standing, in sternal recumbency or in left or right lateral recumbency and can be successfully done via blind palpation of the urinary papilla or through the use of a speculum and light source. In contrast, urinary catheterization for routine purposes (ie, not emergency) is not recommended in cats even with heavy sedation or general anesthesia unless there are unusual circumstances.

For traumatic catheterization, male and female dogs under heavy sedation or general anesthesia are positioned and prepped (as outlined previously); however, the

---

Box 2
Cystocentesis (ultrasound guided, manual palpation and immobilization, blind)

For: culture (best), routine screening, fresh cell morphology for neoplasia (random timing)

Localization: kidneys, ureters, urinary bladder, reproductive tract (retrograde ejaculation in male patients)

Advantages: quick, minimally invasive, least prone to contamination

Disadvantages: requires sufficiently filled bladder, clean and disease-free skin, and personnel trained in sterile techniques. Potential for blood contamination, acute collapse (vagal stimulation).[5] Contraindicated in patients with coagulopathy, thrombocytopenia, anticoagulant therapy, or known bladder neoplasia (seeding). Blind technique: challenging in overweight/obese animals, incidental enterocentesis, and severe hemorrhage (aortic puncture).[5,6]

sample technique is different. Depending on the catheter design, the tip may be cut off or cut at an angle to allow enhanced collection of desired cells. If a large mass is noted along the dorsal wall of the urinary bladder via ultrasound, then the sterile catheter can be wedged up against the wall of the urinary bladder and then repetitively pushed back and forth into the mass. Before this occurs, however, typically a small amount of sterile saline is flushed through the length of the catheter to allow better collection of cells during aspiration. With the sterile syringe attached to the urinary catheter, the catheter is moved back and forth along the mass to try to traumatize the tissue to collect cells and fluid is aspirated repeatedly during this time.[7] The sample typically appears slightly cloudy with saline and tissue/cells present in the sterile syringe, which can then be submitted for cytology. Then, the urinary catheter is gently removed. Although this procedure can be done blindly (can be considered when disease is known to be diffuse), it is possible to traumatize normal urinary bladder tissue rather than obtain samples from the mass. Alternatively, this can be done with cystoscopy guidance to obtain a more directed sample because the mass or abnormal tissue can be visualized in real time. Although this technique can be used to obtain a diagnostic sample for conditions, such as transitional cell carcinoma, it is important to remember that this tissue is not normal; it can be friable and prone to rupture (**Box 3**).

QUALITY ASSURANCE

The method of collection should be associated with the specific sample and documented in the medical record to allow full consideration when interpreting results. Urine pH may increase with storage and, as a result, crystals may form and cellular morphology quickly deteriorates. It is recommended that urinalysis and slide preparations are performed as soon as possible after collection and ideally within 30 minutes.[1] If this is not possible, the urine should be refrigerated for no more than several hours, then rewarmed to room temperature prior to testing. Do not freeze urine intended for microscopic examination (**Box 4**).

EQUIPMENT, PREPARATION, AND HANDLING FOR IN-HOUSE EVALUATION

A basic standard operating procedure is provided **Box 5** and more specific guidelines are available.[1] Laboratorians may elect to use a water-soluble stain to aid examination of cellular elements. If this is done, it should be added to the sediment before it is

---

Box 3
Catheterization (atraumatic and traumatic)

For: assessing known urinary tract infection (antibiotic selection), especially if failure of other methods; urinary tract trauma, neoplasia, or obstruction

Localization: urinary tract (F), urogenital tract (M); previously visualized mass (dogs, traumatic for cytology sample acquisition)

Advantages: Light/no sedation (M); eliminates potential gastrointestinal and reproductive sources of pathology (F)

Disadvantages: requires trained personnel and sterile techniques. Heavier sedation (F). Iatrogenic hemorrhage; not for evaluating hematuria. Not recommended for assessing animals prone to recurrent urinary tract infections unless concurrent urinary tract infection is being evaluated. Potential for infection or urethral or bladder rupture leading to strictures and uroabdomen.[8]

Abbreviations: F, female; M, male.

Box 4
Quality assurance/documentation protocols

- Label containers (not lids): date and time of collection, patient identification.
- Label slide preparations: date of collection, patient identification, sample source (eg, traumatic catheterization), sediment.
- Medical record/report: collection method, sample date and time, personnel.
- Sample handling: test within 30 minutes of collection or refrigerate and rewarm.
- Sediment: refrigerate in small sealed container.

---

resuspended to minimize dilution of the aliquot to be examined. Note, however, that use of such stains may confound interpretation if they contain an overgrowth of bacteria or fungal elements or precipitate that may mimic bacteria. For these reasons, a drop of stained and unstained sediments should be evaluated side by side for more accurate assessment of the microscopic findings.

A technique for sediment examination is summarized in **Box 6**. Results are reported semiquantitatively in a standardized fashion.[1]

CELL MORPHOLOGY AND INTERPRETATION

Neutrophils are probably the most common leukocytes observed in urine; however, lymphocytes, monocytes/histiocytes, and eosinophils also may be present. Familiarity with peripheral blood features is helpful in wet mount identification. Cellular size vary depending on the cell type, concentration or pH of the urine, age of the sample, and presence of bacterial products. Generally, leukocytes are 10 μm to 14 μm (1.5–2 times the size of erythrocytes) and spherical (**Fig. 1A**). Granularity varies with the type of leukocyte present. In some cases, lobulation of neutrophil nuclei may be visible. Typically none to only a few (0–3/high-power field) leukocytes are present in healthy individuals when urine is obtained by cystocentesis. Slightly higher numbers may be observed in sample collected by other means owing to periurethral contamination. Pyuria beyond these circumstances indicates inflammation and/or infection. Differentials for inflammation include infection whether or not organisms are visible, calculi, irritation, and neoplasia. Urine sediment samples can be stained with Romanowsky-type stains to visualize cells and infectious organisms more clearly (see **Fig. 1B**).

Erythrocytes are smaller than leukocytes measuring approximately 5 μm to 7 μm in diameter. They are anucleated cells that range from pink to colorless and round, biconcave, or crenated, depending on the pH, freshness, and concentration of the sample (**Fig. 2**). Crenated erythrocytes may be present in hypertonic or aged urine and can be mistaken for leukocytes because the spicules may be interpreted as

---

Box 5
Urine sediment wet mount preparation

- Centrifuge a 5-mL aliquot of mixed urine at low speed (eg, 450 × g) for 3 to 5 minutes.
- Decant all but 0.5 mL of supernatant and gently resuspend the sediment.
- Place a drop of sediment on a glass slide.
- Apply a no. 1, 22-mm × 22-mm cover slip and allow preparation to settle.
- Evaluate at 100× and 400× magnification for inflammatory or neoplastic cells and bacteria.

Box 6
Urine sediment wet mount examination

- Use microscope of sufficient quality to allow resolution of bacteria with 40× objective.
- The 40× objective indicates the thickness in mm (eg, 0.17) of the appropriate cover slip (no. 1).
- Lower the condenser and/or partially close the condenser diaphragm to enhance contrast.
- Examine the entire sample with 10× (100× total magnification) objective to identify the larger epithelial cells, cell clusters, and casts.
- Examine multiple fields with the 40× (400× total magnification) objective to identify inflammatory cells, erythrocytes, smaller epithelial cells, and organisms.
- Constant focusing with the fine adjustment knob is necessary because wet mounts are dynamic preparations and elements may be in multiple planes of focus.
- Use standardized semiquantitative categories for recording the average number of leukocytes or erythrocytes (eg, none, 0–3, 3–6, 6–10, 10–30, 30–50, 50–100, 100–250, >250) per field and yeast, bacteria, or squamous epithelial cells (eg, none, few, moderate, or many).
- Report the type (rods and/or cocci) and arrangement (pairs/chains) of bacteria.

---

granules. Erythrocytes may be present in low numbers in normal individuals (0–5/high-power field), as a result of iatrogenic contamination related to collection techniques or as a result of pathology related to hemorrhage, inflammation, infection, or neoplasia. Hemorrhage can occur with trauma or necrosis. Note that erythrocytes lyse in hypotonic (urine specific gravity test <1.005) urine.

Epithelial cells may be squamous, transitional, or renal cells. It is recommended that epithelial cells be routinely categorized as squamous and nonsquamous, given the difficulty in accurately distinguishing renal from transitional epithelial cells.

Squamous epithelial cells are large (30–60 μm) flat cells with abundant clear cytoplasm and distinct polyhedral borders (**Fig. 3**). The cells may be anucleated or contain small round to oval nucleus. Some cells may be folded. These are considered contaminants that arise from the distal reproductive tract in female patients or distal urethra. They may also be observed as a result of skin contamination during cystocentesis.

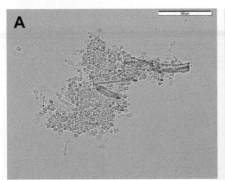 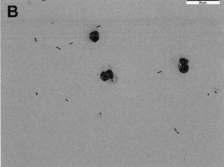

Fig. 1. (*A*) Leukocytes in urine from a cat clustered around debris (wet mount, original magnification ×200). (*B*) Neutrophils in urine from a cat with extracellular and intracellular rod-shaped bacteria (Wright-Giemsa stain, original magnification ×1000).

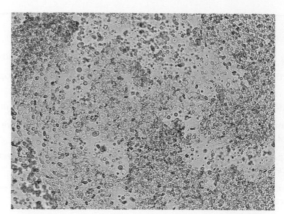

Fig. 2. Many erythrocytes in urine (wet mount, original magnification ×400).

Transitional epithelial cells line the urinary tract from the ureters and bladder through the upper urethra. They range in shape and size, depending on where they originate within the mucosal surface. Those arising from the basilar layer are smaller (approximately 20 μm) and cuboidal to columnar. Those from the intermediate layer are more rounded to caudate and approximately 30 μm whereas those arising from the surface are approximately 40 μm and flattened and more polygonal. As with any epithelial tissue, transitional cells are shed as a result of normal cell turnover and, therefore, may be present in urine in low numbers. These may be shed in higher numbers and exhibit reactive or dysplastic features as a result of irritation and inflammation (**Fig. 4**A). Morphologic features of reactivity and dysplasia are in a continuum with those of malignancy; there is no single criterion that distinguishes the 2. Criteria of malignancy include variation in cell size (anisocytosis), nuclear size (anisokaryosis), nucleolar size and shape, and the presence of mitotic figures, particularly if they are atypical (see **Fig. 4**B, C). Other features might include nuclear or cell molding and multiple nuclei or nucleoli. The more criteria of malignancy that are present, the more confident in making a diagnosis of neoplasia, particularly if there is minimal to no evidence of inflammation. Corroborating information, such as a mass lesion observed in the trigone area, can add to the level of diagnostic confidence. Although transitional cell carcinoma is the most common urinary tract neoplasia, lymphoma and renal cell

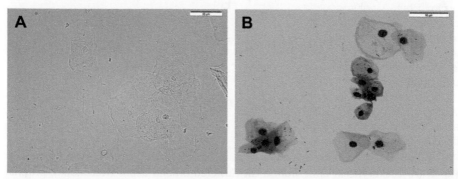

Fig. 3. Squamous epithelial cells ([A] wet mount, original magnification ×400, and [B] Wright-Giema stain, original magnification ×500).

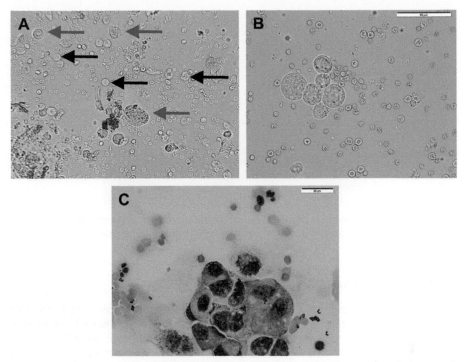

Fig. 4. (*A*) A few transitional cells (*red arrows*) and leukocytes (*black arrows*) and many erythrocytes in urine from a cat, some of which are crenated (wet mount, original magnification ×400). (*B*) Urine from a dog with bladder masses and urinary tract infection. Transitional epithelial cells exhibit criteria of malignancy including anisocytosis and anisokaryosis. Many erythrocytes (often crenated) and occasional leukocytes are also present (wet mount, original magnification ×400). (*C*) Same urine as in (*B*) (Wright-Giemsa stain, original magnification ×1000).

carcinoma are also possible. Suspicious cytologic samples should be sent for confirmation by a clinical pathologist.

Renal epithelial cells originate from the renal tubules and may be found in low numbers because they may be shed in health as a result of normal cell turnover. They tend to be round to oval, range in size from 10 μm to 50 μm, and may have a cytoplasmic tail. A columnar shape with 1 flattened surface of microvilli suggests they came from the proximal tubules. They may be observed singly or in rows. If present in high numbers or incorporated into casts, they indicate renal tubular pathology, such as pyelonephritis or necrosis; however, distinguishing renal tubular cells from leukocytes and transitional epithelial cells can be challenging. Cytologic examination of stained preparations can be helpful.

The presence of spermatozoa has no clinical implications when observed in a voided urine sample from intact male patients. High numbers may suggest retrograde ejaculation in catheterized or cystocentesis samples.[2] These are generally easily identified by the spatulate head and long fine tail (**Fig. 5**). Sperm in fresh samples may be motile. If observed in urine from a female patient, however, verify that the sample was obtained from the appropriate animal and that it was labeled appropriately before informing the owner that the animal was recently bred. Disrupted spermatozoa may be misinterpreted as yeast (heads), long rod-shaped bacteria, or fungal hyphae (tails).

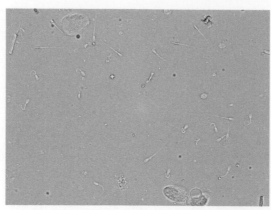

Fig. 5. Urine from an intact male dog. Several spermatozoa are present along with a few transitional epithelial cells and a calcium oxalate crystal (wet mount, original magnification ×400).

COMMON MICROORGANISMS

Bacteria, yeast, and fungi may be present in urine as the result of contamination during collection or staining, or with infection of the bladder or kidneys. Visualization of bacteria in urine sediment requires a microscope with a resolution capable of distinguishing smaller (.38 μm–.72 μm) organisms at 400× magnification. Contaminants arise during collection from the skin or mucosal surface of vaginal areas (voided samples) or gut (accidental enterocentesis during cystocentesis) and they may multiply to significant numbers in urine stored at room temperature. Overgrowth may also occur if the stain becomes contaminated by touching bottle droppers or slides to nonsterile surfaces. Bacterial overgrowth can be minimized by refrigerating stored urine and periodically cleaning staining jars, replenishing with fresh stain, keeping stain jars covered when not in use, and prohibiting the use of the same stain set for fecal smears.

The shape, size, and arrangement of bacterial organisms vary with the type of bacteria present and at least their shape and semiquantitative number should be reported, for example, moderate rods. Random jiggling of small particles, known as brownian motion, is the result of the effects of heat produced from the microscope lamp. For this reason, very small crystals are sometimes misinterpreted as cocci-shaped bacteria because they appear to be alive. Truly motile organisms swim across the field of view. Cocci-shaped bacteria can be present individually or in pairs, chains, and clusters. Because cocci are difficult to distinguish from small crystals and other particles, their presence can be confirmed with Romanowsky staining of an air-dried preparation (**Fig. 6**). The elongate shape of rod-shaped bacteria is more readily identified. Rods may be present individually or in chains (**Fig. 7**). Large rods in chains should be distinguished from fungal hyphae, which are considerably larger and often segmented. Yeast, such as *Candida* sp, are 2 μm to 7 μm × 3 μm to 8 μm spherical to egg-shaped organisms that may be individualized or in the process of budding (**Fig. 8**A). They tend to have a more well-defined border than erythrocytes. With overgrowth, *Candida* form pseudohyphae, which are approximately 3 μm × 10 μm to 15 μm with septae-like constrictions between segments (see **Fig. 8**B). Lipid droplets are quite round and often float in a higher plane whereas yeast settles (see **Fig. 8**C). True hyphae observed with invasion of mucosal surfaces are narrower and longer without segmentation.[9]

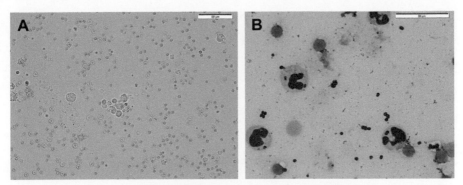

Fig. 6. (*A*) Cocci-shaped bacteria arranged in small clusters are barely visible. Many erythrocytes, a few leukocytes, occasional transitional epithelial cells and one hyaline cast are also present (wet mount, original magnification ×400). (*B*) Cocci are readily visible intracellularly and extracellularly when stained (Wright-Giemsa stain, original magnification ×1000).

ANCILLARY TESTS AND SHIPPING CONSIDERATIONS FOR CLINICAL PATHOLOGY CONSULTATION

Because biochemical constituents and crystal types and number may change and cells in whole urine do not retain morphology in stored urine, sending whole urine for evaluation is not advised unless the referral center can receive the sample within a short time after collection. The type of sample submitted for confirmation varies somewhat with the formed element that is in question. Centrifuge the urine and submit only the sediment resuspended in 0.5 mL of urine in a small, sealed container for general review of the entire sediment or crystal identification. Refrigerate the sample during storage and shipping. Because cellular morphology is not retained in whole urine, organisms can die or multiply, and wet mounts do not provide sufficient detail, films for cytologic evaluation should be made as soon as possible after sample collection.

If there are formed elements, such as suspicious cells or organisms, observed in the wet mount prep, further evaluation can be done on air-dried and Romanowsky-stained films. Two techniques are summarized in **Box 7** and demonstrated in **Fig. 9**. Leukocytes stain as observed in blood films, crystals tend to be faint if at all visible, and bacteria and yeast can be observed using a 100× oil objective and stain dark purple.

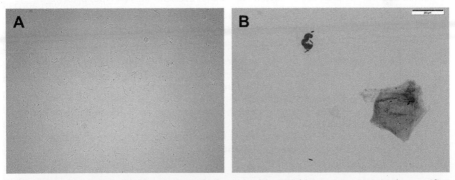

Fig. 7. (*A*) Many rod-shaped bacteria with three leukocytes (wet mount, original magnification ×400). (*B*) A leukocyte with intracellular rod-shaped bacteria and one squamous epithelial cell (Wright-Giemsa stain, original magnification ×1000).

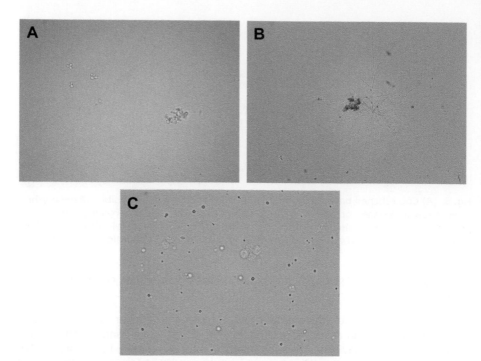

Fig. 8. (*A*) Budding yeast, consistent with *Candida* spp and 2 hyaline casts (wet mount, original magnification ×400). (*B*) Urine containing a mat of fungal pseudohyphae and many cocci in the background (wet mount, original magnification ×100). (*C*) Urine with a few leukocytes and variably sized lipid droplets in different planes of focus (wet mount, original magnification ×400).

Box 7
Urine cytology film preparation

- Remove coverslip from the wet mount prep and air dry. Stain with Romanowsky-like (quick) stain to confirm the presence of bacteria or further evaluate the cell types present.

- If the presence of bacteria is confirmed, a second preparation can be made from the sediment, which is air dried, heat fixed, and Gram stained to determine Gram-staining characteristics.

- If cells are too rounded or ruptured, further cellular detail is desired, or if there are cells suspicious for neoplasia, recentrifuge sediment, decant, and gently resuspend supernatant. Make 2 pull/squash preps on remaining sediment.
  - Place a drop of gently resuspended sediment on each of 2 glass slides adjacent to the label end. Gently place the 2 slides on top of each other, drops to the inside, and quickly pull the 2 slides in opposing directions.
  - If resistance is felt, the cells have probably been ruptured. Attempt another preparation with larger drops and/or quicker movements.

- (Quick) stain one to evaluate for intact cells.

- If cells are ruptured, prepare additional films using a larger drop and/or quicker pull technique, air dry, stain one, and evaluate, as described previously.

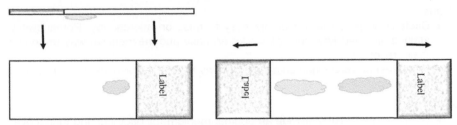

Fig. 9. Pull (or squash) prep to make 2 films simultaneously.

Intracellular bacteria indicate infection rather than contamination. This also provides a better means of evaluating transitional and renal epithelial cells.

Gram staining should only be performed after the presence of bacteria is confirmed by morphology (rods) or Romanowsky staining (cocci). Gram staining results may be unreliable, however, owing to the viability and type of the bacteria as well as whether the sample was over-decolorized or under-decolorized. Alternatively, a recently marketed test with a high sensitivity, specificity, and positive and negative predictive values for detecting Gram-positive and Gram-negative bacteria in urine (Rapid-Bac Vet, Silver Lake Research Corporation, Monrovia, CA) is commercially available.[10]

Despite described limitations, urine samples collected via a voided sample can be submitted for culture and sensitivity but the colony-forming units (CFU)/mL are required for interpretation. A voided urine sample from a dog containing less than 10^5 CFU/mL of bacteria is not considered clinically significant.[11] If greater than or equal to this number of bacterial counts is present, however, a cystocentesis, if not medically contraindicated, is recommended to confirm the presence of an infection. The presence or absence of clinical signs, predisposing conditions for infection, whether there is concurrent pyuria and the type of bacteria grown in culture must also be considered.[12] Sample handling recommendations for quantitative culture are available at microbiology laboratories and online.[1]

Urine fungal antigen tests may be warranted in cases suspected of systemic fungal infections, such as histoplasmosis or blastomycosis.[13,14]

A bladder tumor antigen test performed on urine has been shown sensitive and specific in dogs with transitional cell carcinoma without concurrent urinary tract disease. It is not specific, however, if there is concurrent pyuria, bacteriuria, or hematuria.[15,16]

If a pathologist's evaluation is warranted, send both the Romanowsky-stained and air-dried unstained and unfixed films (see **Box 7**; **Box 8** for helpful hints).

A recently marketed automated sediment analyzer (IDEXX Laboratories, One IDEXX Drive Westbrook, ME) claims the ability to evaluate 45 fields on a few drops of urine within a few minutes for blood and epithelial cells, bacteria, casts, and common crystals. A peer-reviewed validation of this product has yet to be published.

Box 8
Shipping hints for sediment and film review

- Ship urine sediment in small, tightly sealed container (eg, bullet tube) overnight with a cold pack.
- Ship a stained and unstained sediment film for pathologist review if cells suspicious for neoplasia, such as transitional cell carcinoma, are present.
- Do not freeze, heat fix, or expose films to formalin fumes, temperature extremes, or condensation.

Pearls
- Bacteria, in particular cocci, are easy to miss on microscopy. Romanowsky-stained air-dried sediment allows for an easy and inexpensive way to confirm their presence.
- Rapid test strips provide an alternative way to detect presence as well as Gram characteristics of urine.

Pitfalls
- Contaminated stains provide an optimal medium for bacterial and fungal overgrowth. Be sure to use separate staining jars for fecal and ear samples and clean jars and replace stain regularly.
- Cells do not preserve well in urine. Send freshly prepared concentrated films when requiring a pathologist's evaluation of the cellular elements.

SUMMARY

The focus of this article is on the cytologic examination of urine sediment for evidence of inflammation, infection, and/or neoplasia. Methods of sample collection and handling play a critical role with interpretation of results and are described. Proper film preparation is also important whether evaluating in house or submitting for a pathologist's review, and several techniques are provided. The images demonstrate the utility of appropriate film preparation and staining to maximize cytologic evaluation.

REFERENCES

1. Gunn-Christie RG, Flatland B, Friedrichs KR, et al. ASVCP quality assurance guidelines: control of preanalytical, analytical, and postanalytical factors for urinalysis, cytology, and clinical chemistry in veterinary laboratories. Vet Clin Pathol 2012;41(1):18–26.
2. Beaufays F, Onclin K, Verstegen J. Retrograde ejaculation occurs in the dog, but can be prevented by pre-treatment with phenylpropanolamine: a urodynamic study. Theriogenology 2008;70(7):1057–64.
3. Forrester SD, Grant DC. Cystocentesis and urinary bladder catheterization. In: Ettinger SJ, Feldman EC, editors. Textbook of veterinary internal medicine. 7th edition. Saunders Elsevier; 2010. p. 432–3.
4. Lulich JP, Osborne CA. Cystocentesis: lessons from thirty years of clinical experience. In North American Veterinary Community clinician's brief. Urology. Available at: http://www.cliniciansbrief.com/sites/default/files/sites/cliniciansbrief.com/files/cystocentesis.pdf. Accessed April 27, 2016.
5. Odunayo A, Ng ZY, Holford AL. Probable vasovagal reaction following cystocentesis in two cats. J Feline Med Surg Open Rep 2015;1(1):1–4. Available at: http://jor.sagepub.com/content/1/1/2055116915585021.full. Accessed April 27, 2016.
6. Buckley GJ, Aktay SA, Rozanski EA. Massive transfusion and surgical management of iatrogenic aortic laceration associated with cystocentesis in a dog. J Am Vet Med Assoc 2009;235(3):288–91.
7. Morrison WB. Instruments and techniques for nonsurgical biopsy. In: Roantree CJ, editor. Cancer in dogs and cats: medical and surgical management. 2nd edition. Jackson (WY): Teton NewMedia; 2002. p. 118.
8. Stafford JR, Bartges JW. A clinical review of pathophysiology, diagnosis, and treatment of uroabdomen in the dog and cat. J Vet Emerg Crit Care (San Antonio 2013;23(2):216–29.

9. Sudbery Peter E. Growth of Candida albicans hyphae. Nat Rev Microbiol 2011;9: 737–48.
10. Jacob ME, Crowell MD, Fauls MB, et al. Diagnostic accuracy of a rapid immuno-assay for point-of-care detection of canine urinary tract infection. Am J Vet Res 2016;77(2):162–6.
11. Labato MA. Uncomplicated urinary tract infection. In: Bonagura JD, editor. Kirk's current veterinary therapy XIV. Philadelphia: Elsevier Health Sciences; 2009. p. 918–21.
12. Smee N, Loyd K, Grauer G. UTIs in small animal patients: part 1: etiology and pathogenesis. J Am Anim Hosp Assoc 2013;49(1):1–7.
13. Spector D, Legendre AM, Wheat J, et al. Antigen and antibody testing for the diagnosis of blastomycosis in dogs. J Vet Intern Med 2008;22(4):839–43.
14. Foy DS, Trepanier LA, Kirsch EJ, et al. Serum and urine blastomyces antigen con-centrations as markers of clinical remission in dogs treated for systemic blasto-mycosis. J Vet Intern Med 2014;28(2):305–10.
15. Billet HG, Moore AH, Holt PE. Evaluation of a bladder tumor antigen test for the diagnosis of lower urinary tract malignancies in dogs. Am J Vet Res 2002;63(3): 370–3.
16. Henry CJ, Tyler JW, McEntee MC, et al. Evaluation of a bladder tumor antigen test as a screening test for transitional cell carcinoma of the lower urinary tract in dogs. Am J Vet Res 2003;64(8):1017–20.

Common Infectious Organisms

Craig A. Thompson, DVM[a],*, Amy L. MacNeill, DVM, PhD[b]

KEYWORDS

- Cytology • Cytopathology • Fungi • Bacteria • Infectious • Canine • Feline

KEY POINTS

- Cytology is a useful tool to identify a variety of lesions, ranging from immune-mediated to degenerate, neoplastic, and inflammatory.
- Careful attention to the cytomorphologic details of the organism in conjunction with lesion location and signalment allows for their identification.
- Rapid diagnosis of an infectious etiology allows for a rapid institution of therapy, thus maximizing prognosis for a given case.

INTRODUCTION

Lesions have many types of etiologies and can affect every tissue in the body. Cytopathology is an extremely useful tool that can be used to identify lesions and their etiologies. Regardless of the method of sample acquisition (ie, fine needle aspiration [FNA], impression, scraping, or body cavity effusion aspiration), obtaining samples for cytologic evaluation generally induces less morbidity compared with obtaining samples for histologic evaluation (ie, incisional biopsy or excisional biopsy). Indeed, some tissues such as body cavity effusions, cerebrospinal fluid, and peripheral blood are not tissues that can be easily examined via histology. In addition to being easier to obtain, cytopathologic evaluation of tissues is much quicker compared with histologic evaluation of tissues. The need for cumbersome and expensive tissue processing and staining makes histology a diagnostic modality relegated to a diagnostic laboratory, whereas the entire process of acquisition, processing, and evaluation of cytology samples can be entirely performed within a practice. All of these features make cytology the ideal tool to quickly and accurately identify infectious agents as the

The authors have nothing to disclose.
[a] Clinical Pathology, Department of Comparative Pathobiology, College of Veterinary Medicine, Purdue University, 725 Harrison Street, West Lafayette, IN 47907-2027, USA; [b] Clinical Pathology, Department of Microbiology, Immunology, and Pathology, College of Veterinary Medicine and Biomedical Sciences, Colorado State University, 300 West Drake Road, Fort Collins, CO 80523-1644, USA
* Corresponding author.
E-mail address: cathomps@purdue.edu

etiology of a lesion, providing the practitioner a way to begin treatment essentially immediately.

This article discusses a few common infectious organisms that can be clearly identified cytologically. Several infectious agents can be identified cytologically, but require additional diagnostic techniques (eg, culture) to speciate the organism. Some organisms are not infectious in immunocompetent animals, but have been isolated from lesions in immunosuppressed animals. Examples of organisms reported to cause infection in immunosuppressed dogs are listed in **Table 1**.

FUNGI

Fungal infections can induce morbidity and mortality in veterinary patients. Culture of fungal agents can take weeks and pose a risk of infection to laboratory personal.[1] Although the discovery of serologic tests has vastly improved the diagnosis of and monitoring of some fungal infections,[2] cytologic visualization still offers an immediate diagnosis.

Blastomycosis

Blastomycosis is caused by the dimorphic fungus *Blastomyces dermatitidis*. Canine disease is much more likely than feline; however, unlike dogs, who frequently obtain infections from the outside environment, feline cases have been identified in strictly indoor animals.[3] Lesions, and thus samples, associated with blastomycosis often are from the lung, skin, or lymph nodes. These can take the form of direct lung aspirates, transtracheal washes (TTWs), or bronchoalveolar lavages (BALs) as well as FNA of nodes and nodules or swabs from draining skin lesions. Less frequently obtained lesions include those from the orbit, bone, and prostate. Less common locations include the testes, bladder, brain, mammary gland, and synovial joints. Suppurative to pyogranulomatous inflammation is commonly associated with infection,[4–6] frequently with necrotic debris scattered about. Neutrophils are nondegenerate to apoptotic. The round yeast itself is generally not difficult to locate, depending on the tissue examined (**Table 2**). They range in size from 10 to 40 μm and have a thick blue wall (**Fig. 1**). They can be seen budding in a broad-based fashion, with the daughter cell being nearly as large as the parent (**Fig. 2**). Fungal organisms, including *Blastomyces spp* stain positive with periodic acid–Schiff (PAS) stain (**Fig. 3**).

Histoplasmosis

This systemic fungal disease is caused by the dimorphic fungus *Histoplasma capsulatum*. Samples that are commonly used to diagnose histoplasmosis include the lungs (BAL, TTW), lymph nodes, spleen, rectum, bone marrow, gastrointestinal (GI) tract, body cavity effusion, and peripheral blood. Cats tend to have more respiratory signs and lesions, whereas dogs show more GI signs.[7–9] Inflammatory patterns vary; however, the inflammation that is often associated with histoplasmosis lesions is

Table 1
Infectious disease agents reported in immunosuppressed dogs

Protozoal	Bacterial	Viral	Fungal
Acanthomoeba spp	Actinomycetes	Herpesvirus	*Cokeromyces recurvatus*
Toxoplasma spp	*Bartonella spp*	Adenovirus	Phaeohyphomycoses
	Mycoplasma spp	Distemper virus	*Phialosimplex caninus*
	Nocardia spp.	Papillomavirus	*Pneumocystis (carinii) jiroveci*

Table 2
Different tissues sampled and the frequency of identifying organism in dogs infected with *Blastomyces dermatitidis*

Cytologic Sample	Reference Number 5/6	Number Positive (%) 5/6
Lung aspirate	57/16	46 (81)/4 (25)
TTW	39/14	27 (69)/4 (29)
Sputum	4	4 (100)
Lymph node	24/54	19 (79)/36 (67)
Skin	32/46	31 (97)/39 (85)
Prostate	3	3 (100)
Eye	3/5	2 (67)/5 (100)
Joint	2	2 (100)

macrophagic to somewhat granulomatous. The yeast itself is round and measures 3 to 5 μm and has a colorless cell wall with a dark interior (**Figs. 4–6**). They are often found clumped within macrophages and infrequently free (from lysed cells) in the background.

Cryptococcosis

Another systemic disease caused by a dimorphic fungus, cryptococcosis is caused by *Cryptococcus sp*. Cytologic specimens include cerebrospinal fluid (CSF), skin nodules, nasal exudate, and a variety of other sites; however, the organism is most frequently observed in CSF samples.[10] Organisms were observed in 66% and 55% of cats and dogs, respectively, in one retrospective study.[10] This organism is unusual in that the inflammatory response associated with it ranges from essentially no inflammation to marked inflammation. Likewise, although known for its large, nonstaining capsule, some variants have no perceptible capsule at all. That being said, when present, the inflammatory response is typically macrophagic to some degree, often with eosinophils. The organism itself ranges in size from 8 to 40 μm and is round in shape with a slightly thickened wall and dark interior (**Fig. 7**). It can be seen replicating by

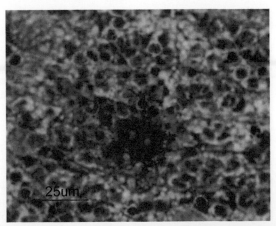

Fig. 1. Two *Blastomyces* spherules on top of a thick background of suppurative inflammation. Note the thick blue wall and broad based budding. Modified Wright, 1000×.

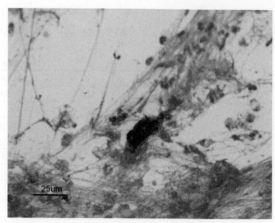

Fig. 2. Broad-based budding *Blastomyces* in a moderate background of necrotic debris. 60×
Modified Wright, 600×.

narrow-based budding (**Fig. 8**). The capsule of *Cryptococcus* is colorless and non-staining (traditional stains) and can reach up to 200 μm in diameter. No-encapsulated forms exist and can mimic other fungi such as *Blastomyces spp* or be missed completely unless a high index of suspicion is present. Staining with PAS can help identify the organism (**Fig. 9**).

Sporotrichosis

Sporotrichosis is an infection generally confined to the skin and mucocutaneous areas of dogs, with cats also showing clinical signs of infection elsewhere, including lung and the GI tract. The disease is caused by *Sporothrix schenckii*. It is of distinct importance, as it is generally regarded to as a zoonotic disease. Samples obtained for cytopathologic examination often come from skin lesions such as raised lesions and ulcerated, open wounds. Cytologically, the presentation is marked inflammation with numerous intralesional yeast. Diagnostic accuracy in cats has been demonstrated to be 82.8% in

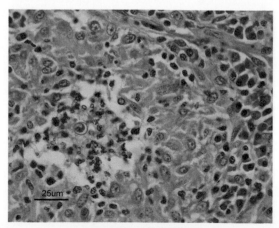

Fig. 3. A single *Blastomyces* spherule in the middle of dense, pyogranulomatous inflammation. PAS, 600×.

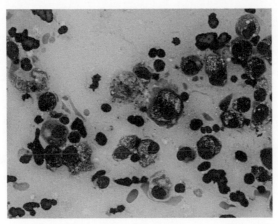

Fig. 4. Feline lung aspirate. Multiple foamy macrophages are noted. Rarely within macrophages and free in the background are a few round *Histoplasma* organisms. Diff-Quik. 600×.

a study involving 244 cats.[11] Organisms were observed in 76% of the exudative lesions from 44 dogs in another study.[12] The yeasts are oval to round, budding organisms that measure 3 to 5 μm by 5 to 9 μm and are mainly seen within macrophages and neutrophils, occasionally free in the background (**Fig. 10**). Inflammatory patterns are usually mixed to pyogranulomatous.

Aspergillosis

Sinonasal aspergillosis is caused most frequently by *Aspergillus fumigatus*; however, *A niger, A nidulans,* and *A flavus* have also been implicated. These other species are morphologically and clinically indistinguishable. Positive samples are often obtained via rhinoscopy or rhinotomy and often involve necrotic tissue and/or fungal plaques.

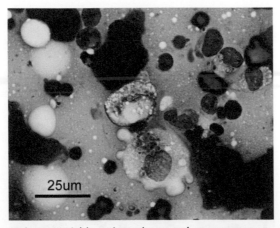

Fig. 5. Feline liver aspirate. Variably activated macrophages among several darkly staining hepatocytes. The macrophages often contain several yeast. These yeast are also rarely seen free in the background. Diff-Quik. 1000×.

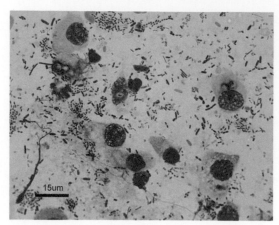

Fig. 6. Canine rectal scrape. Two yeast spherules seen within a mononuclear cell with 2 spherules free in the background along with the medium-sized, mixed population of bacteria. Diff-Quik. 1000×.

Occasionally nasal discharge or direct nasal swabbing can produce diagnostic samples, although not as successfully.[13] If inflammation can be identified, it tends to be macrophagic to mixed to pyogranulomatous. The fungal hyphae are septate (every 2–8 μm), and exhibit dichotomous branching at 45° angles (**Figs. 11** and **12**). To add to the cytologic obfuscation, the hyphae themselves are variably staining, often poorly to nonstaining, using traditional polychromatic stains. The hyphae can be highlighted by using special stains, PAS, or a silver stain, such as Gomori methenamine silver (GMS, **Fig. 13**). These stains are particularly useful when a high index of suspicion exists, and hyphae cannot be seen among the necrotic debris.

Dermatophytosis

Dermatophytes may cause skin lesions in many mammals including dogs, cats, and people. Lesions typically appear as an alopecic, red ring on the skin, which contributes

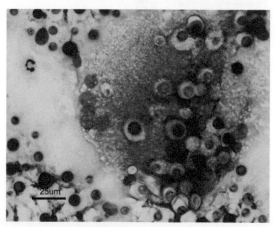

Fig. 7. Abundant encapsulated organism seen, many within a large, foamy macrophage. Modified Wright. 1000×.

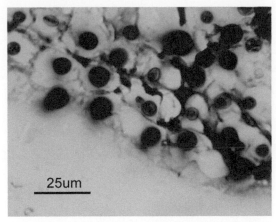

Fig. 8. A solid mat of encapsulated organisms without inflammation. Note the narrow based budding in the center of the photomicrograph. Modified Wright. 1000×.

to the name of the disease, ringworm. Dermatophytosis is most commonly diagnosed by culture of the organism, but organisms may be observed microscopically on a skin scraping. Numerous spores from the organism are the most likely component of the organism to be detected cytologically. Spores are small (1–3 μm in diameter), round, and have a thin clear capsule (**Fig. 14**). They are often found extracellularly and are associated with suppurative inflammation.

BACTERIA

All types of bacterial organisms are easily diagnosed cytologically if enough of the organisms are present in the lesion. It is best to collect samples from lesions that are likely infected with bacteria before administration of antibiotics, as even inappropriate antibiotic treatment may reduce the number of bacterial organisms present and prevent detection of the organisms using cytology. In lesions that contain bacteria, it is

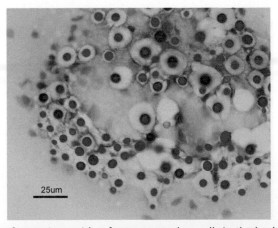

Fig. 9. Heavy mat of organisms with a few mononuclear cells in the background. Note the variable thickness of the capsule. PAS. 1000×.

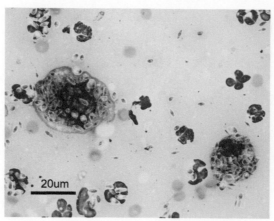

Fig. 10. Abundant round- to oval-shaped organisms are seen filling 2 macrophages and occasional neutrophils, with many free in the background. Modified Wright. 1000×.

important to determine if the organisms are a contaminant or commensal organism within the sample, or if they are pathogenic. Extracellular bacteria are likely to be contaminants or commensal organisms. However, when bacteria are observed within inflammatory cells, they are considered pathogenic. Most infectious bacterial cocci and rods are found within neutrophils. The neutrophils usually have a degenerate appearance with swollen, pale nuclei. There are a few types of bacteria that tend to be observed within macrophages instead of neutrophils; two of these organisms are discussed in more detail below.

Bacterial pathogens may be the primary cause of the lesion or may be a secondary infection induced by an underlying disease process. Additional clinical and cytologic findings are used to distinguish primary from secondary bacterial infections. Another important aspect is whether a single bacterial morphology is detected cytologically or a mixed bacterial population is seen. This can directly affect treatment decisions. For example, the antibiotic treatment that is most appropriate for infection with a bacterial coccus is different than the antibiotic treatment most appropriate for a bacterial rod. A

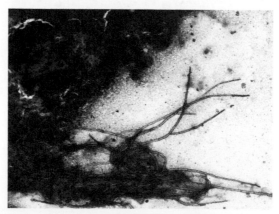

Fig. 11. Mat of tangle fungal hyphae with abundant, amorphous necrotic debris. Diff-Quik. 1000×.

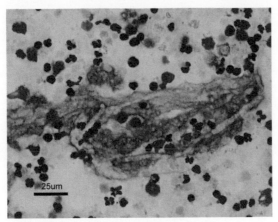

Fig. 12. Kidney aspirate, dog. Negative-staining hyphae can be seen admixed within the nuclear debris and suppurative inflammation. Diff-Quik. 1000×.

mixed bacterial population in an abdominal effusion is another critically significant cytologic finding; this provides evidence for leakage of intestinal contents and is an indication for immediate surgical exploration.

Cellular and stain debris can easily be misinterpreted as bacterial organisms. Bacteria are typically uniform in appearance. They are 1 μm in width and stain blue with Romanowsky stains such as Diff-Quik. By definition, bacterial cocci are round, and rods are elongated. Although detection of bacteria in a lesion is a useful finding. More specific information about bacterial organisms often requires additional stains, culture of the organism, antibiotic sensitivity testing, serum titers, or molecular techniques (such as polymerase chain reaction [PCR] assays). However, there are a few bacterial organisms that are more specifically identified by cytology alone.

Mycobacterium spp

Mycobacterium spp are gram-positive, acid-fast staining rod-shaped bacteria that cause a wide range of clinical syndromes, depending on the location of the lesion(s).

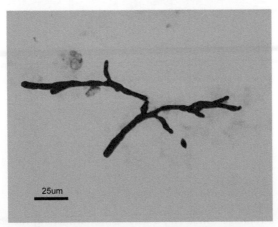

Fig. 13. Same case as **Fig. 12**. Hyphae stain black with GMS. 1000×.

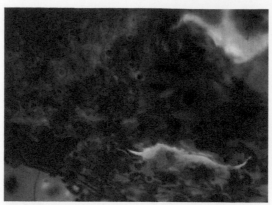

Fig. 14. Skin scraping, cat. Small fungal spores with a thin clear capsule are closely associated with suppurative inflammation. Wright-Giemsa. 1000×.

Similarly, a wide range of species has been implicated in disease including *M avium*, *M tuberculosis* complex (MTBC), and *M bovis*. Marked pyogranulomatous inflammation is the most common finding, regardless of tissue involved. Using routine polychromatic stains, the organism appears as nonstaining filamentous rods within macrophages (**Fig. 15**).

Neorickettsia helminthoeca

In canine patients that live in or visit the Pacific Northwest, *Neorickettsia helminthoeca* should be a differential diagnosis in dogs with acute fever, ocular discharge, vomiting, depression, and diarrhea. Lymph nodes are typically enlarged in patients with *N helminthoeca*, and the organism can be identified by FNA of the nodes. The organism typically causes granulomatous lymphadenitis and can be detected within macrophages as small, variably shaped, roughly 1 to 2 μm diameter, basophilic inclusion bodies (**Fig. 16**).

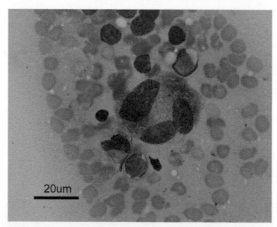

Fig. 15. Solitary macrophage containing a few faint, nonstaining rod-shaped organisms. Modified Wright. 1000×.

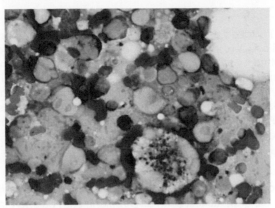

Fig. 16. Lymph node aspirate, dog. One large macrophage containing neorickettsial inclusion bodies is shown among many, variably sized lymphocytes. Wright-Giemsa. 1000×. (*Courtesy of* Dr M. Elena Gorman, Oregon State University, Corvallis, OR.)

Actinomyces/Nocardia

Filamentous bacteria are considered pathogenic when present in an inflammatory lesion, even if intracellular organisms are not observed. *Actinomyces spp* and *Nocardia spp* are filamentous bacteria that are morphologically similar in cytologic appearance and can cause similar diseases. Generally regarded as pyogenic, the inflammation they incite can progress to pyogranulomatous. In addition to lesions in solid tissues, they have also been implicated in 15% to 19% of culture-positive pyothoraces.[14] The organisms are long, filamentous rods that have a beaded appearance and often taper at the ends (**Fig. 17**). Occasionally, clumps/colonies of organism will form, often referred to as sulfur granules. This is a feature more often seen with *Actinomyces spp*.

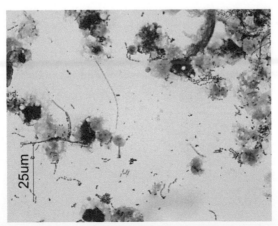

Fig. 17. Direct smear thoracic effusion. A mixed population of bacteria is observed, including a long, beaded rod with slightly tapered ends. Modified Wright. 1000×.

PROTOZOA

There are several protozoal diseases of significance in dogs and cats including giardiasis, cryptosporidiosis, toxoplasmosis, and babesiosis. *Cytauxzoon felis* is a protozoal organism transmitted by ticks that causes severe illness in cats. Clinical signs of disease are nonspecific and include fever, lethargy, anorexia, and weakness. Piroplasms can be identified readily within erythrocytes on a peripheral blood smear. Piroplasms are 1 to 2 μm in diameter and round with a pinpoint, eccentrically located nucleus and clear cytoplasm (**Fig. 18**). The organism has been reported throughout the Southeast and in parts of the Midwest.[15]

PARASITES

GI parasites are commonly detected microscopically by visualizing eggs in wet mount samples of feces. Other parasites, such as *Dirofilaria spp*, can be detected in peripheral blood. Microfilaria are also occasionally seen in cytologic samples as a contaminant from peripheral blood. *Dirofilaria spp* are nematode parasites are transmitted via mosquito vectors. *Dirofilaria immitis* is the causative agent of heartworm disease. Larvae can be visualized microscopically in peripheral blood of affected dogs. Larvae have a slightly tapered head and have a pointed tail. They are approximately 300 μm in length and 6 μm in width (**Fig. 19**). The larvae can be detected microscopically using many laboratory techniques including preparation of direct blood smears, smears of plasma following centrifugation of the blood, Knott test, and filter tests.

VIRAL

It is not possible to identify most viral infections using cytology alone; however, viral diseases that form inclusion bodies in infected cells can be identified. Examples of these include poxviruses (eg, cowpox virus), herpesviruses, adenoviruses, and paramyxoviruses (eg, morbillivirus) infections. Canine distemper virus is a morbillivirus that may be detected in peripheral blood cells on a direct blood smear and epithelial cells from conjunctival swabs. Viral inclusions formed by distemper virus are cytoplasmic, rounded, and have a smooth or glassy appearance (**Fig. 20**). Note that the apparent color of viral inclusions may vary with different cytologic stains.

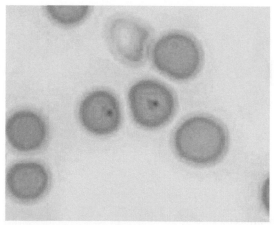

Fig. 18. Peripheral blood smear, cat. Small piriform-shaped *Cytauxzoon felis* organisms can be seen within erythrocytes. Wright-Giemsa. 2000×.

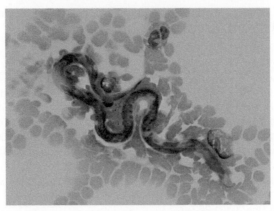

Fig. 19. Peripheral blood smear, dog. A large microfiliarial organism is shown. The head is slightly tapered, and the tail is sharply pointed, consistent with *Dirofiliaria immitus*. Wright-Giemsa. 1000×.

SUMMARY

This article was meant to give a brief overview of some common infectious organisms that can be identified cytologically in lesions of dogs and cats. Although cytology can provide relatively specific information about pathogens, even more commonly, it identifies general infectious causes of disease, allowing clinicians to begin the patient on an effective treatment regimen almost immediately. In short, cytology is a powerful

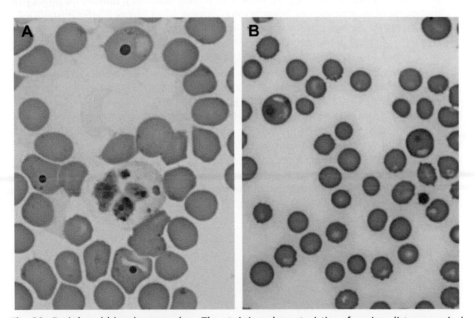

Fig. 20. Peripheral blood smear, dog. The staining characteristics of canine distemper viral inclusions vary with different types of cytologic stains. (*A*) Viral inclusions appear bright purple to fuchsia when stained with Diff-Quik stain. (*B*) Viral inclusions look dark purple to blue when stained with Wright Giemsa. 2000×.

tool that can be used to diagnose infectious etiologies quickly and reliably, with reasonable sensitivity and high specificity.

REFERENCES

1. Singh K. Laboratory-acquired infections. Clin Infect Dis 2009;49(1):142–7.
2. Spector D, Legendre AM, Wheat J, et al. Antigen and antibody testing for the diagnosis of blastomycosis in dogs. J Vet Intern Med 2008;22(4):839–43.
3. Blondin N, Baumbardner DJ, Moore GE, et al. Blastomycosis in indoor cats: suburban Chicago, Illinois, USA. Mycopathologia 2007;163(2):59–66.
4. Garma-Avina A. Cytologic findings in 43 cases of blastomycosis diagnosed antemortem in naturally-infected dogs. Mycopathologia 1995;131(2):87–91.
5. Crews LJ, Freeney DA, Jessen CR, et al. Utility of diagnostic tests for and medical treatment of pulmonary blastomycosis in dogs: 125 cases (1989–2006). J Am Vet Med Assoc 2008;232(2):222–7.
6. Arceneaux KA, Taboada J, Hosgood G. Blastomycosis in dogs: 115 cases (1980-1995). J Am Vet Med Assoc 1988;213(5):658–64.
7. Aulakh HK, Aulakh KS, Troy GC. Feline histoplasmosis: a retrospective study of 22 cases (1986-2009). J Am Anim Hosp Assoc 2012;48(3):182–7.
8. Mitchell M, Stark DR. Disseminated canine histoplasmosis: a clinical survey of 24 cases in Texas. Can Vet J 1980;21(3):95–100.
9. Brömel C, Sykes JE. Histoplasmosis in dogs and cats. Clin Tech Small Anim Pract 2005;20(4):227–32.
10. Trivedi SR, Sykes JE, Cannon MS, et al. Clinical features and epidemiology of cryptococcosis in cats and dogs in California: 93 cases (1988-2010). J Am Vet Med Assoc 2011;239(3):357–69.
11. Jessica N, Sonia RL, Rodrigo C, et al. Diagnostic accuracy assessment of cytopathological examination of feline sporotrichosis. Med Mycol 2015;53(8):880–4.
12. Schubach TM, Schubach A, Okamoto T, et al. Canine sporotrichosis in Rio de Janeiro, Brazil: clinical presentation, laboratory diagnosis and therapeutic response in 44 cases (1998-2003). Med Mycol 2006;44(1):87–92.
13. De Lorenzi D, Bonfanti U, Masserdotti C, et al. Diagnosis of canine nasal aspergillosis by cytological examination: a comparison of four different collection techniques. J Small Anim Pract 2006;47(6):316–9.
14. Walker AL, Jang SS, Hirsh DC. Bacteria associated with pyothorax of dogs and cats: 98 cases (1989–1998). J Am Vet Med Assoc 2000;216(3):359–63.
15. MacNeill AL, Barger AM, Skowronski MC, et al. Identification of *Cytauxzoon felis* infection in domestic cats from southern Illinois. J Feline Med Surg 2015;17(12): 1069–72.

Index

Note: Page numbers of article titles are in **boldface** type.

A

Actinomyces/Nocardia, 161
Acute leukemia, 61–63
Anal sac adenocarcinoma
   cytology of, 92
Apocrine gland tumors
   cytology of, 91–94
Arthrocentesis
   sequential
      synovial fluid analysis with, 115
Aspergillosis, 155–156

B

Bacteria, 157–161
   Actinomyces/Nocardia, 161
   introduction, 157–159
   Mycobacterium spp., 159–160
   Neorickettsia helminthoeca, 160
Basilar epithelial tumors
   cytology of, 88–89
B-cell chronic lymphocytic leukemia (CLL)
   cytology and flow cytology correlates related to, 58–59
Benign lytic lesions
   of bone
      cytology of, 82
Bicavitary effusions
   in retrospective study of canine peritoneal fluid analysis, 128
Blastomycosis, 152
Bone(s)
   aspiration of, 72–73
   cytology of, **71–84**
      benign lytic lesions, 82
      described, 73
      introduction, 71
      neoplasia, 77–81
      osteomyelitis, 74–76
      vs. histopathology, 71–72
   reactive, 73–74
Bone marrow aspirate
   evaluation of, **31–52**
      bone marrow smear preparation and, 34–35

Vet Clin Small Anim 47 (2017) 165–174
http://dx.doi.org/10.1016/S0195-5616(16)30115-2
0195-5616/17

Printed and bound by CPI Group (UK) Ltd, Croydon, CR0 4YY

07/10/2024

01040502-0017